The Agentic Department

A Blueprint for the Future of Medical Imaging

From Implementation Life Cycles to General Medical Intelligence (2026–2030)

DR. BASEM GARADA

COPYRIGHT

The Agentic Department: A Blueprint for the Future of Medical Imaging

From Implementation Life Cycles to General Medical Intelligence (2026–2030)

Published by **Digi Health Services, LLC**.

First Edition: 2026

Printed in the United States of America.

CLINICAL & LEGAL DISCLAIMER

Purpose and Scope

The information presented in *The Agentic Department* is for educational and strategic planning purposes only. It is intended to provide a visionary framework for the integration of agentic AI in medical imaging. This text does not constitute medical advice, legal counsel, or a definitive clinical protocol.

The "Human-in-the-Loop" Mandate

In the agentic era, all AI-driven outputs—including but not limited to autonomous triage alerts, automated anatomical measurements, and drafted radiology reports—must be treated as probabilistic suggestions. The human physician remains the Final Accountable Party. Clinical decisions, informed by a patient's unique history and physical examination, must always supersede algorithmic reasoning. No AI agent possesses the ethical or legal authority to make a final diagnostic or therapeutic decision without human validation.

AI-Assisted Content Disclosure

This manuscript was developed with the assistance of generative AI tools to support research organization, structural logic, and drafting refinement. Every clinical conclusion, technical specification, and ethical guideline has been independently curated, reviewed, and verified by the author. The final content reflects the author's professional expertise and editorial responsibility.

Liability and Risk

The field of medical AI is rapidly evolving. While every effort has been made to ensure the accuracy of the 7-Phase Lifecycle and modality-specific benchmarks, the author and publisher disclaim any liability for adverse clinical outcomes, financial losses, or security breaches resulting from the implementation of technologies discussed herein. Readers are advised to consult with local regulatory bodies (FDA, NIST, etc.) and hospital legal counsel before initiating any agentic shift.

ACKNOWLEDGEMENTS

The creation of this blueprint, and the broader vision of **Digi Health Services**, has been made possible through the collaboration, dedication, and shared foresight of many individuals across the clinical, technical, and administrative landscapes.

First and foremost, I would like to extend my deepest gratitude to the **Frontline Clinical Teams**—the radiologists, technologists, sonographers, and nurses. You are the "Human Guardrails" of medicine. Your willingness to adapt to new workflows and your tireless commitment to patient safety provided the real-world data and feedback loops that transformed theoretical algorithms into practical, agentic partners.

To the **Engineering and Data Science Teams at Digi Health Services**: Thank you for your relentless pursuit of interoperability. By championing and implementing global standards like FHIR, DICOMweb, and the Model Context Protocol, you have built the "Digital Nervous System" that allows our agents to reason, communicate, and serve. You have turned the abstract promise of AI into a tangible reality for the clinicians and patients who depend on us.

I am also profoundly grateful to the **Hospital Administrators and Policy Makers** who recognized that the transition to an Agentic Department is not merely a capital expense, but a strategic investment in the future of human health. Your courage to pilot these systems in "Shadow Mode" and your commitment to ethical AI governance have set a global standard for the industry.

A special thanks to my **Mentors and Peers** in the radiological community. Our debates on the "Renaissance of the Physician" and the risks of skill atrophy were essential in shaping the balanced, critical perspective of this book. You reminded me that while the technology is exciting, the mission is—and always will be—the patient.

Finally, to my **Family**, whose patience and support allowed me the time to document this journey. Your belief in the mission of Digi Health Services has been my greatest source of inspiration.

This book is dedicated to those who see beyond the pixels to the people they represent.

— Dr. Basem Garada

FOREWORD

In the early decades of the twenty-first century, we were promised that technology would simplify medicine. Instead, we witnessed the "Great Digital Friction." For every advance in imaging resolution, there was a corresponding increase in physician burnout. For every new data point, there was a new administrative burden. We became masters of the pixel, yet slaves to the interface.

I founded Digi Health Services on a singular, defiant premise: technology should not be a weight we carry, but a partner that carries the weight for us.

For too long, the conversation around Artificial Intelligence in healthcare has been trapped in a binary of fear and hype. We were told AI would either replace the radiologist or simply serve as a glorified spell-checker. Both perspectives were too narrow. The true revolution is not about "detection"; it is about agency.

As we enter 2026, we are witnessing the birth of the Agentic Department. This is an ecosystem where intelligence is no longer passive. It is a world where agents reason, collaborate, and execute—allowing the physician to step away from the keyboard and return to the bedside.

This book is the culmination of years of clinical practice, technical integration, and a deep-seated belief that the future of medicine is human-centric, powered by machine-autonomy. Within these pages, I offer you a blueprint—a structured, engineering-led roadmap to transition your department from a state of reactive exhaustion to one of proactive excellence.

The "Agentic Shift" is not a luxury for the future; it is a necessity for the present. We owe it to our patients, and we owe it to ourselves, to build a healthcare system that is as smart as the people who work within it.

Welcome to the new era of medical imaging.

— Dr. Basem Garada

Founder & CEO, Digi Health Services, LLC

January 2026

Table of Contents

INTRODUCTION: THE AGENTIC SHIFT

The field of medical imaging has spent the last decade in a state of "AI anticipation." We have seen thousands of algorithms cleared by the FDA, millions of dollars invested in point solutions, and endless debates about the eventual replacement of the radiologist. Yet, as we enter 2026, the reality on the ground has revealed a different truth: the challenge was never about the algorithm's ability to "see" a lesion—it was about the system's ability to act.

Welcome to the era of **The Agentic Department**.

For years, artificial intelligence in radiology functioned like a sophisticated spell-checker—passive, narrow, and disconnected. Today, under the leadership of Digi Health Services, we are architecting an ecosystem of Autonomous Agents. These are not mere tools; they are dynamic entities that possess the ability to reason across modalities, navigate complex EHR workflows via FHIR, and collaborate with clinical teams in real-time.

A Note on the 2026 Perspective

This book is written from a "near-future" vantage point. The case studies and "Digi Health Insights" found within these chapters are visionary narratives designed to stress-test our current technological trajectory. While the specific patient scenarios are fictional, the underlying architectures—such as Agentic Orchestration and Physics-Informed Reasoning—represent the real-world roadmap we are currently building. These "fictional" examples serve as the North Star for what a fully realized Agentic Department will achieve.

"The Agentic Department: A Blueprint for the Future of Medical Imaging" is designed to be the definitive manual for this transition. We move beyond the "if" and "when" of AI to the how.

In the following chapters, we will explore:

- **The Technical Foundation:** How the Model Context Protocol (MCP) and multimodal transformers allow agents to speak a common language.
- **The Implementation Life Cycle:** A rigorous, 7-phase approach to deploying intelligence across every imaging modality, from the high-velocity world of CT to the sterile, real-time environment of Interventional Radiology.
- **The Human Interface:** Defining the new roles of the "Future Doctor"—the physician who no longer just reads images, but orchestrates a symphony of digital experts.

As the founder of Digi Health Services, my goal with this blueprint is to provide a pragmatic, ethical, and highly efficient roadmap. We are not just upgrading our software; we are redesigning the social contract of healthcare. We are building a future where technology handles the complexity, so that the clinician can return to the core of their calling: the patient.

The scanners are humming. The agents are waiting for their instructions. It is time to begin.

— Dr. Basem Garada

SECTION I

FOUNDATIONS AND FRAMEWORKS

CHAPTER 1: THE SILICON CATALYST – AI AND THE MODERN REVOLUTION

The Dawn of the Cognitive Era

The 21st century will not be remembered merely for its digital connectivity, but for the fundamental shift in the nature of intelligence itself. If the Industrial Revolution of the 18th century provided the "muscle" to automate physical labor, the Artificial Intelligence (AI) revolution of the 21st century provides the "neural tissue" to automate and augment cognition. We are currently living through a period of transition that parallels the discovery of electricity—a general-purpose technology that does not just improve one specific industry, but fundamentally rewires the architecture of human civilization.

To understand where we are going in the specialized field of medical imaging, we must first understand the ocean in which we are swimming. AI is no longer a niche subfield of computer science relegated to academic laboratories; it has become the primary engine of global innovation. Since the turn of the millennium, and specifically following the "Deep Learning explosion" of 2012, AI has transitioned from rule-based systems—where humans had to manually program every "if-then" scenario—to self-learning architectures that identify patterns within data that remain invisible to the human eye.

From Logic Gates to Neural Networks

The evolution of AI since the year 2000 has been characterized by three converging forces: the exponential increase in computational power, the explosion of "Big Data," and the refinement of sophisticated algorithms. In the early 2000s, AI was largely predictive and narrow. We saw it in the recommendation engines of early e-commerce and the spam filters of our email inboxes. These were "Narrow AI" systems—tools designed to perform a single task at a level comparable to or slightly better than a human.

However, the revolution truly accelerated with the advent of Artificial Neural Networks (ANNs). By mimicking the layered structure of the human brain, specifically through Deep Learning, we granted machines the ability to "see" and "hear." This shift transformed AI from a tool of calculation into a tool of perception. In the last decade alone, we have witnessed the mastery of Natural Language

Processing (NLP), allowing machines to converse with nuance, and Computer Vision, allowing machines to interpret visual stimuli with a precision that often exceeds human capability.

A Multi-Industry Disruption

Before we narrow our lens to the clinical environment, we must acknowledge how AI has already revolutionized other sectors of humanity. This cross-industry implementation provides the blueprint for the medical advancements we will discuss in later chapters.

- **Finance and Global Markets:** In the financial sector, AI agents manage trillions of dollars in assets. They detect fraudulent transactions in milliseconds, identifying anomalies that would take a human auditor weeks to uncover. High-frequency trading algorithms respond to global news cycles faster than a human can blink, stabilizing (and sometimes disrupting) markets with mathematical coldness.

- **Transportation and Logistics:** The dream of the autonomous vehicle is perhaps the most visible manifestation of AI's impact on humanity. By integrating LiDAR, computer vision, and real-time sensor fusion, AI is redefining the concept of mobility. Beyond self-driving cars, AI optimizes global supply chains, predicting demand surges and rerouting shipping lanes to ensure the global economy remains fluid.

- **Energy and Sustainability:** AI is being used to manage smart grids, predicting energy consumption patterns to reduce waste. In climate science, AI models process petabytes of satellite data to track deforestation and carbon emissions, providing humanity with the data-driven insights needed to fight ecological collapse.

- **Creative Arts and Communication:** The recent rise of Generative AI has challenged our very definition of "creativity." From generating photorealistic images to composing complex code and literature, AI has moved from being a passive observer to an active creator.

The Shift from Tools to "Agents"

Crucially, we are moving away from seeing AI as a static tool and toward seeing it as an Agent. This is a distinction that will be central to this book. While a "tool" requires constant human input to produce an output, an "agent" possesses a degree of autonomy. It can perceive its environment, reason about the best course of action to achieve a goal, and execute that action.

In the context of the 21st century, the AI agent is the ultimate collaborator. It does not just provide a result; it participates in the workflow. As we move into the second and third sections of this book, we will explore how these agents act not just as "calculators for X-rays," but as active participants in the diagnostic journey, assisting clinicians in navigating the overwhelming deluge of medical data.

The Moral and Philosophical Weight

The revolution of AI is not without its frictions. As AI begins to permeate every facet of human life, it brings with it profound questions of ethics, bias, and agency. If an AI agent makes a decision, who is responsible? How do we ensure that the algorithms are fed diverse data so they do not replicate human prejudices? These questions are not merely academic; in the medical field, they are matters of life and death.

As we conclude this introduction to the general landscape of AI, it is important to view this technology as a mirror. AI reflects our collective knowledge, our data, and our desires. It is a catalyst that amplifies our capabilities. For the medical professional, the implementation of AI across other industries serves as both a roadmap and a warning. We have seen how AI can streamline efficiency and uncover hidden truths, but we have also seen the necessity of "Human-in-the-loop" systems.

Looking Toward the Medical Horizon

With this foundation established, we can see that AI is not a fleeting trend. It is the new infrastructure of human thought. The transition of AI into the medical industry—and specifically into the highly specialized world of medical imaging—is the logical next step in this evolution. In the following chapters, we will peel back the layers of general AI to focus on its most profound application: the preservation and enhancement of human health through the digital eye.

CHAPTER 2: THE MEDICAL METAMORPHOSIS – AI IN THE HEALTHCARE ECOSYSTEM

The Crisis of Capacity

The modern healthcare system is currently facing a "perfect storm." Across the globe, we are witnessing a demographic shift: an aging population with increasingly complex chronic conditions is placing an unprecedented strain on a workforce that is itself shrinking. It is projected that by 2030, the global health workforce shortage will reach 10 million providers. This is not merely a staffing issue; it is a capacity crisis.

Simultaneously, we have entered the age of "Medical Big Data." A single patient today is no longer just a physical body; they are represented by terabytes of digital information—electronic health records (EHRs), high-resolution genomic sequences, pharmacy histories, and real-time streams from wearable sensors. For a human clinician, the sheer volume of this data has surpassed the "cognitive limit." When a physician spends more time interacting with a keyboard than with a patient, the system is fundamentally broken. AI is no longer a luxury for futuristic research; it is the necessary "operating system" required to manage the complexity of 21st-century medicine and return the focus to human-to-human care.

The Four Pillars of AI in Medicine

To understand how AI is reshaping this ecosystem, we can categorize its impact into four foundational pillars:

- **Pillar I: Precision Diagnostics**
  Diagnostics has historically been an exercise in human pattern recognition. However, AI—specifically machine learning—can detect "sub-perceptual" patterns. In oncology, AI models can analyze pathology slides or dermatological images to identify cellular irregularities that are invisible to the naked human eye. This is not about replacing the doctor, but about providing a "super-lens" that enhances the threshold of what can be detected, leading to earlier intervention and drastically better survival rates.

- **Pillar II: Personalized Treatment (The "N-of-1" Model)**

Traditional medicine often relies on "population-based" evidence—what works for the average person. AI allows us to pivot toward "Personalized Medicine." By synthesizing a patient's genetic markers with their environmental data and medical history, AI agents can predict which specific medication or dosage will be most effective for that unique individual. This reduces the dangerous "trial-and-error" phase that currently plagues treatments for cancer, mental health, and autoimmune diseases.

- **Pillar III: Administrative Autonomy**
  Perhaps the most immediate relief for the healthcare workforce comes from administrative AI. Natural Language Processing (NLP) models now act as "ambient scribes," listening to a doctor-patient conversation and automatically generating a structured medical note. By automating the "drudgery" of billing, scheduling, and coding, AI agents act as an invisible administrative layer that frees up hours of a clinician's day, directly combating the global epidemic of physician burnout.

- **Pillar IV: Drug Discovery and Genomics**
  The "bench-to-bedside" pipeline—the process of bringing a new drug to market—traditionally takes over a decade and billions of dollars. AI is radically shortening this timeline. Models like AlphaFold have already solved 50-year-old challenges in protein folding, allowing researchers to simulate how drugs will interact with the body before a single molecule is synthesized in a lab. This acceleration is crucial for reacting to emerging pathogens and treating rare genetic disorders that were previously considered "unprofitable" to research.

Current Implementation Benchmarks (2024–2026)

As we move through 2026, we are seeing these theories turn into standard clinical protocols. We have moved past the "pilot phase."

- **The Triage Revolution:** In modern Emergency Departments, AI now works as a first-line triaging tool. When an MRI or CT scan is completed, an algorithm scans it in seconds for "red-flag" conditions like an acute stroke or a pulmonary embolism. If detected, the case is automatically moved to the top of the radiologist's queue, saving precious minutes that equate to saved brain tissue or lives.

- **Predictive ICU Analytics:** Critical care units now utilize "Early Warning Systems" that monitor heart rate, blood pressure, and oxygen levels in real-time. These systems can predict a septic event or a cardiac crash up to six hours before a human nurse would see the physical symptoms, allowing for preemptive intervention.

Barriers to Entry: The "Trust Gap"

Despite the technological prowess of AI, its integration into the clinical ecosystem is often met with resistance. This resistance is not born of a fear of change, but rather of a fundamental "Trust Gap" that persists between the silicon and the stethoscope.

- **The Black Box Problem:** At the heart of this distrust is the issue of explainability. Deep learning models, by their nature, are opaque. They can process millions of data points to conclude that a patient is at high risk for a cardiovascular event, but they often cannot explain *why*. In a field where the "gold standard" is evidence-based reasoning, a "black box" that says "trust me" is often unacceptable. As we move into 2026, the focus is shifting toward Explainable AI (XAI)—systems designed to show their "reasoning" via heatmaps or feature-weighting, allowing clinicians to validate the logic behind the machine's suggestion.

- **Data Silos and Interoperability:** AI is only as good as the data it consumes. Historically, medical data has been trapped in proprietary, non-standardized formats. For AI to be truly effective, it requires seamless Interoperability. This means that the AI must be able to pull data from a patient's wearable heart monitor, their local GP's notes, and the hospital's high-resolution imaging archives simultaneously. Without universal data standards like FHIR (Fast Healthcare Interoperability Resources), AI remains a fragmented tool rather than a cohesive partner.

- **The Regulatory Labyrinth:** The FDA and other global bodies have had to invent a new category of oversight: Software as a Medical Device (SaMD). Unlike a physical scalpel or a drug, AI is "living" software that updates and evolves. Regulating a moving target requires a "lifecycle-based" approach where the AI is continuously audited for safety and bias, long after its initial release.

Ethical Considerations: Bias and Accountability

The implementation of AI in medicine raises profound ethical questions that humanity is only beginning to answer.

- **Algorithmic Bias:** If an AI is trained on data primarily from one demographic, its accuracy may plummet when applied to another. We have already seen instances where AI diagnostic tools for skin cancer were less accurate on darker skin tones due to a lack of diversity in training sets. Ensuring Equity in AI is a primary mandate for developers in this new era.

- **The Accountability Vacuum:** If an AI agent recommends a treatment that leads to a complication, who is responsible? Is it the developer who wrote the code, the hospital that deployed it, or the doctor who followed its advice? The current consensus is the "Human-in-the-loop" (HITL) model, which dictates that AI should augment, not replace, human judgment. The AI provides the insight; the human provides the accountability.

Transition: From Passive Tools to Active Agents

As we conclude this chapter, we must recognize a fundamental shift occurring right now. Most of what we have discussed so far involves "Passive AI"—tools that sit and wait for a human to ask them a question or upload a file.

However, we are standing on the precipice of a new paradigm: Agentic AI.

Unlike a passive tool, an AI Agent has a degree of autonomy. It does not just wait for an image to be uploaded; it actively monitors the incoming stream of images, cross-references them with the patient's history, alerts the relevant specialist, and potentially even schedules a follow-up appointment before a human has even walked into the reading room. In the next chapter, we will narrow our focus to the core of this book: how these autonomous agents are specifically revolutionizing the world of Medical Imaging.

CHAPTER 3: THE ARCHITECTURE OF AN AGENT – DEFINING THE DIGITAL COLLEAGUE

The Critical Distinction: Tool vs. Agent

To the casual observer, an AI "tool" and an AI "agent" might look the same—both involve software processing medical data. However, the architectural difference is as vast as the difference between a traditional map and a self-driving car.

- **The AI Tool (Passive):** This is reactive. It requires a human to "trigger" it. For example, a radiologist opens a chest CT and manually clicks a button to run a nodule detection algorithm. The tool provides a result and then stops. It has no memory of the patient's previous scans and no ability to communicate its findings beyond the local screen.

- **The AI Agent (Active):** This is goal-oriented and proactive. It operates on a continuous loop of Perception, Reasoning, and Action. An agent does not wait for the radiologist; it monitors the hospital's "worklist" in real-time. If it sees a new CT scan, it autonomously fetches the patient's history, compares the new image to scans from three years ago, and—if it finds a change—alerts the oncology team directly while drafting a preliminary report.

The Four Pillars of Agentic Architecture

For a system to be classified as an "Agent" in medical imaging, it must possess four core architectural modules:

I. Perception (The Multimodal Eye)

In the context of this book, perception goes beyond simple image recognition. An imaging agent uses Multimodal Perception. It "sees" the pixels of an MRI, but it also "reads" the clinical indication in the referral note and "interprets" the patient's recent lab results (e.g., creatinine levels before injecting contrast). It merges these different data streams into a single "contextual vector" to understand *why* the image was taken.

II. Memory (The Longitudinal Context)

A major flaw in early medical AI was its "amnesia." Every scan was treated as a brand-new event. Agentic architecture includes:

- **Short-term Memory:** Keeping track of the current diagnostic steps.
- **Long-term Memory:** Utilizing "Vector Databases" to store and retrieve a patient's historical imaging trends. This allows the agent to say, "This lesion hasn't just appeared; it has grown by 2mm since 2024."

III. Reasoning and Planning (The Cognitive Core)

This is where the agent decides *how* to solve a problem. If an agent detects an ambiguous mass on an ultrasound, its "reasoning engine" (often powered by a Large Language Model or a specialized Vision-Language Model) might decide that the most logical next step is to recommend a follow-up MRI. It "plans" the diagnostic pathway rather than just flagging a pixel.

IV. Action (The Integrated Hand)

An agent must be able to affect the world. In a radiological workflow, "Action" means:

- Automatically "pre-fetching" relevant old studies.
- Populating a draft report in the RIS (Radiology Information System).
- Sending a high-priority "ping" to a surgeon's mobile device for critical findings like an intracranial hemorrhage.

Multi-Agent Systems (MAS): The Digital Radiology Team

The future of medical imaging does not rely on one "super-AI," but rather on a Multi-Agent System. In this book, we will explore how different specialized agents collaborate:

- **The Triage Agent:** Manages the queue and prioritizes urgent cases.
- **The Modality Agent:** Specialized in a specific type of scan (e.g., a "Stroke Agent" for CT or a "Lesion Agent" for MRI).
- **The Communication Agent:** Ensures the findings reach the right human at the right time in the right format.

SUMMARY OF SECTION I: THE FOUNDATIONAL SHIFT

In this opening section, we have traced the evolution of artificial intelligence from a computational curiosity to the essential infrastructure of modern medicine. We have established that the "Agentic

Shift" is not merely a technological upgrade, but a necessary response to a healthcare system at its breaking point.

- **The Catalyst: In Chapter 1**, we identified AI as a "General Purpose Technology" on par with electricity. We explored the transition from rule-based programming to self-learning neural networks, establishing that the power to automate cognition is the defining catalyst of our era.

- **The Metamorphosis: In Chapter 2**, we analyzed the "Crisis of Capacity." We moved beyond the hype to see how AI provides the four pillars—Precision, Personalization, Administration, and Discovery—required to rescue clinicians from "data fatigue" and return them to the bedside.

- **The Digital Colleague: Finally, in Chapter 3**, we defined our protagonist: the Autonomous Agent. We differentiated these proactive, reasoning entities from the passive, narrow tools of the last decade. We established the architecture of the "Digital Colleague"—one that understands context, utilizes the Model Context Protocol (MCP), and operates with a degree of agency previously reserved for human staff.

We have now laid the "Silicon Tracks" upon which the rest of this blueprint runs. We have the history, the necessity, and the architectural definitions in place.

As we move into Section II, we leave the theoretical behind. We will step into the imaging suite and examine, modality by modality, how these agents are being deployed on the front lines—from the high-speed throughput of X-ray to the precise, real-time guidance of Interventional Radiology.

The era of passive observation is over. The era of the Agent has begun.

SECTION II

MODALITY-SPECIFIC IMPLEMENTATION

CHAPTER 4: THE FIRST LINE OF DEFENSE – AI AGENTS IN X-RAY IMAGING

Introduction: The High-Volume Challenge

If MRI is the "luxury vehicle" of imaging—slow, detailed, and expensive—then the X-ray is the "workhorse." Globally, billions of radiographs are taken annually. In any busy Level 1 Trauma Center, the X-ray machine never stops; it is the primary tool for diagnosing everything from a child's fractured wrist to a life-threatening tension pneumothorax.

The challenge in X-ray imaging is not just "interpretation," but throughput. Radiologists often face "stacks" of hundreds of chest X-rays, many of which are routine or normal. Within this mountain of data, the "needle in the haystack"—the subtle lung nodule or the faint hairline fracture—can be missed due to cognitive fatigue. Furthermore, the time between a technologist taking an image and a radiologist reading it can range from minutes to hours. In critical cases, this "latency" is the difference between recovery and catastrophe. This is where the X-Ray Agent transforms from a tool into a life-saving colleague.

The X-Ray Agent Architecture: Perception to Action

To implement an AI agent in the X-ray suite, we must apply the four-fold architecture established in Section I.

I. **Perception: The "Point-of-Care" Eye**

In X-ray, the agent's perception begins at the Modality Edge. Modern X-ray agents are increasingly integrated directly into the hardware of the X-ray machine. As soon as the detector captures the photons, the agent "sees" the raw data.

Its first task is Quality Perception. Is the patient rotated? Did the technologist "clip" the top of the lungs? Is there a foreign object (like a necklace) obscuring the anatomy? By perceiving these technical errors in real-time, the agent can prompt the technologist to re-take the image immediately, while the patient is still on the table, preventing the "recall" cycle that wastes time and resources.

II. Memory: The Power of Comparison

An X-ray is rarely a static event; it is a snapshot in a longitudinal timeline. The Digi Health agentic architecture utilizes Longitudinal Memory to transform a single image into a temporal narrative. When a chest X-ray is pushed to the PACS, the agent does not wait for a command; it autonomously utilizes the Model Context Protocol (MCP) to "handshake" with the archive and retrieve relevant prior studies.

Unlike a human clinician, who must manually open, tile, and visually "eye-ball" two separate images, the agent performs a high-precision Pixel-Level Subtraction. It recalls the 2024 scan and aligns it geometrically with the 2026 scan.

By analyzing the delta between these two data sets, the agent's reasoning engine evolves:

- **From Detection to Trend**: If a "patchy opacity" in the right lower lobe has increased in density or volume, the agent does not merely label it "pneumonia." It identifies it as a "progressive infiltrate."

- **Contextual Alerting**: By recognizing this trend, the agent can cross-reference the EHR via FHIRcast to see if the patient is currently on antibiotics. If the infiltrate is progressing despite treatment, the agent escalates the case as a "Potential Treatment Failure," providing the clinician with a trend-based insight rather than just a static observation.

III. Reasoning: Contextual Triage

Reasoning in X-ray imaging requires the agent to understand Priority. Using Natural Language Processing (NLP) to read the "Reason for Study" (e.g., "Shortness of breath, rule out PE"), the agent prioritizes its search.

If the agent detects a pneumothorax (a collapsed lung), its reasoning engine recognizes this as a "Critical Finding." It understands that this specific case must bypass the standard chronological worklist. This is not just "detection"; it is operational logic.

IV. Action: Closing the Loop

The "Action" phase is where the agent proves its worth as a teammate. For a positive finding, the agent executes a series of programmed actions:

1. **Worklist Orchestration:** It "paints" the case red in the Radiologist's worklist and moves it to the #1 position.
2. **Reporting Integration:** It pre-populates the "Findings" section of the radiology report with measurements (e.g., "3cm pneumothorax detected in the left apex").
3. **Direct Communication:** It sends an automated, encrypted alert to the referring physician's mobile device, ensuring that the human "loop" is closed within seconds of the image being taken.

Key Clinical Use Cases: From Lungs to Limbs

Chest Radiography (CXR): The "Bread and Butter"

The chest X-ray is the most common and perhaps the most difficult to read perfectly every time. Agentic AI excels here in identifying:

- **Pneumothorax and Pleural Effusion:** High-stakes findings that require immediate drainage.
- **Nodule Detection:** Identifying 5-10mm nodules that might be the earliest signs of lung cancer, often obscured by ribs or heart shadows.
- **Support Device Placement:** In the ICU, agents check if endotracheal tubes, PICC lines, and pacemakers are correctly positioned, alerting the nursing staff if a tube has migrated.

Musculoskeletal (MSK): Precision in Trauma

In orthopedic imaging, agents are used to detect subtle fractures that the human eye might miss, especially in the "dark" hours of a night shift.

- **The "Hidden" Fracture:** Agents are trained to look for cortical irregularities in the scaphoid (wrist) or the femoral neck (hip), where a missed diagnosis can lead to permanent disability or avascular necrosis.

- **Growth Plate Sensitivity:** In pediatric cases, agents act as a "safety net" to distinguish between a normal growth plate (epiphysis) and a true fracture, a common point of confusion for non-specialized clinicians.

Workflow Integration: The "Invisible Assistant"

The goal of the X-Ray Agent is to be **unobtrusive**. It lives "behind the curtain." For the technologist, the agent is an assistant that ensures high image quality. For the radiologist, it is an "extra set of eyes" that never gets tired, never gets hungry, and never has a "bad day."

By automating the routine—the "normals"—the agent allows the radiologist to spend their limited cognitive energy on the most complex and ambiguous cases. In 2026, the implementation of these agents has transitioned from "experimental" to "standard of care" in high-volume centers, reducing the "time-to-report" for critical findings from 4 hours to less than 4 minutes.

To truly understand how an AI agent operates in the X-ray suite, we must look under the hood. In the 2026 landscape, the "magic" of AI has been replaced by robust, standardized technical frameworks. The agent is not just a clever algorithm; it is a highly integrated piece of medical infrastructure.

Technical Implementation: The Infrastructure of Intelligence

The implementation of an X-ray agent generally follows one of two paths: Edge AI (Local) or Cloud-Native AI (Remote). In 2026, the industry has largely settled on a "Hybrid-Edge" model to balance speed with processing power.

Processing at the "Edge"

For X-ray, latency is the enemy. When a technologist is performing a portable chest X-ray in a crowded ER, they cannot wait 60 seconds for a cloud server to return a "quality check."

- **Edge Integration:** The AI agent lives on a specialized GPU (like the NVIDIA IGX Thor or similar medical-grade edge chips) housed directly inside the X-ray generator or the technologist's workstation.

- **Real-Time Feedback:** This allows for "Micro-Latency" processing. The agent analyzes the raw pixels as they are streamed from the detector, providing a "Re-take" alert within 500 milliseconds if it detects motion artifact or suboptimal positioning.

The DICOM and HL7 "Handshake"

Interoperability is the language of the hospital. An agent that cannot "talk" to the rest of the system is a silo.

- **DICOM Structured Reporting (SR):** In the past, AI simply "burned" a red box onto an image. In 2026, agents use DICOM-SR. This allows the agent to send its findings as structured data that the PACS (Picture Archiving and Communication System) can actually "read" and display as interactive overlays.

- **Orchestration:** An "AI Orchestrator" acts as the traffic cop. It uses DICOM Query/Retrieve to fetch historical images for the agent's "Memory" module and employs HL7 FHIR protocols to pull the patient's clinical history (e.g., "History of Lung Cancer") from the Electronic Health Record (EHR).

Limitations and The "Human-in-the-Loop"

As advanced as these agents are, they are not infallible. The technical implementation must include "Guardrails" to prevent the two biggest risks in AI: Automation Bias and The False Positive Burden.

- **The False Positive Burden:** If an agent flags every tiny shadow as a "potential fracture," it creates "alert fatigue." Modern agents utilize a Confidence Threshold—the system only pings the doctor's phone if its confidence score is above 95%. Anything lower is simply highlighted in the report for the radiologist to review at their leisure.

- **Final Verification:** Legally and clinically, the agent is a "Sophisticated Advisor." Every action the agent takes—from drafting a report to flagging a case—must be **validated** by a human radiologist. In Section III of this book, we will discuss the "Review-and-Validate" workflow that has replaced the "Search-and-Type" workflow of the early 2000s.

DIGI HEALTH INSIGHT: The "Ever-Watchful" X-Ray Agent

The Challenge: The Blind Spot of "Satisfaction of Search" A high-volume orthopedic clinic was processing over 200 studies daily. A patient presented for a routine post-operative ankle check following a malleolar fracture repair. The human radiologist, focused on the integrity of the surgical hardware (the primary clinical question), confirmed the hardware was stable. However, a faint, non-displaced fracture in the proximal tibia—located at the extreme periphery of the image—was overlooked due to "satisfaction of search," a common cognitive bias where finding one abnormality leads to the premature ending of the search.

The Agentic Solution: The Digi Health "Geometric Audit" Working silently at the NVIDIA IGX Thor edge layer, the Digi Health X-Ray Agent performed a comprehensive audit in milliseconds, bypassing human cognitive fatigue.

- **Sub-Perceptual Edge Detection:** While the human eye was drawn to the high-contrast metal hardware, the agent's computer vision flagged the cortical irregularity in the proximal tibia, generating a high-confidence heat map for the radiologist's second look.
- **Contextual Correlation via MCP:** Utilizing the Model Context Protocol, the agent autonomously accessed the patient's Biomechanical Digital Twin. It noted a recent bone density score (DEXA scan) indicating significant osteopenia and a clinical history of a "low-energy fall." This multi-modal reasoning made the secondary fracture a high-probability finding rather than a technical artifact.

- **Autonomous Escalation:** Before the patient could leave the clinic and potentially bear weight on the vulnerable limb, the agent triggered an Automated Triage event. It "painted" the case red in the worklist and pushed an encrypted alert to the surgeon's tablet, ensuring immediate stabilization.

Conclusion: The Sentinel at the Edge

The X-ray agent serves as the "First Line of Defense" in the modern imaging department. By combining high-speed edge processing on the NVIDIA IGX Thor platform with a deep, MCP-enabled integration into the hospital's data fabric, it ensures that no critical finding is lost in the noise of a high-volume clinical environment.

We have moved beyond the era where X-ray was a "dumb" modality producing static film. Today, it is a proactive entry point for the Agentic Shift. By automating the "bread and butter" of radiology and providing a layer of digital safety that was technically impossible a decade ago, we do more than just improve diagnostics—we recover the clinician's most valuable asset: time.

As we leave the two-dimensional world of radiography, we turn our attention to a significantly more complex data landscape. In the next chapter, we will explore how these same agentic principles—Perception, Memory, Reasoning, and Action—are applied to the multi-dimensional, high-resolution world of Computed Tomography (CT).

CHAPTER 5: THE MULTI-DIMENSIONAL SHIFT – AI AGENTS IN CT

Introduction: Managing the Data Deluge

If the X-ray is a single snapshot, the modern CT scan is a high-definition feature film. With the mainstream adoption of multi-detector row CT (MDCT) and the arrival of clinical Photon-Counting CT (PCCT) in 2025, the data landscape has shifted fundamentally. A single patient study now generates upwards of 3,000 individual "slices," each containing microscopic levels of spectral data.

For the human radiologist, this creates a massive cognitive bottleneck. The time required to manually scroll through these massive datasets, identify precise anatomical landmarks, and hunt for subtle pathologies is growing exponentially, while the time allotted for patient care remains stagnant. We are asking human eyes to process data at a resolution that exceeds human biology.

The goal of the Digi Health CT Agent is to solve this "Data Deluge" not by looking at images faster, but by understanding them deeper. By moving beyond simple 2D overlays, we have introduced Volumetric Intelligence—a framework where the agent perceives the patient as a continuous 3D entity.

This marks the definitive end of the "slice-by-slice" era. In the Agentic Department, we no longer interpret images in isolation; we analyze volumes in context.

The CT Agent Architecture: 3D Perception and Reasoning

To handle the complexity of CT, the agentic architecture must evolve beyond simple pattern matching.

I. **Perception: 3D Spatial Vision**
   In CT, the agent utilizes Vision Transformers (ViTs) and 3D Convolutional Neural Networks (CNNs). Unlike 2D models, these architectures allow the agent to perceive the patient as a volume. It understands the "spatial hierarchy"—how a lung nodule relates to the pleural surface or how a coronary artery winds through the heart muscle. This volumetric perception is critical for detecting "sub-slice" abnormalities that might be invisible if viewed only in one plane.

II. Memory: Temporal and Structural Continuity

A CT Agent utilizes Longitudinal Memory to solve the most critical clinical question in radiology: *"Is this new?"* In the Agentic Era, we have moved beyond simply tiling old and new images on a screen for visual comparison.

By utilizing Deformable Registration, the agent mathematically overlays a historical scan (e.g., from 2023) with the new 2026 acquisition. This process uses complex warping algorithms to adjust for differences in patient positioning, varied breath-hold volumes, and even post-surgical anatomical changes.

Leveraging the Model Context Protocol (MCP), the agent does not just look at the pixels; it digests the previous narrative. It tracks the exact "doubling time" of a lung lesion or the millimeter-level widening of an aortic aneurysm over years. This provides a high-fidelity Quantitative History—a precise growth-velocity curve that a human eye could only estimate. By turning "stability" from a subjective opinion into a statistical fact, the Agent transforms the CT scan into a predictive tool for long-term patient management.

III. Reasoning: Multimodal Correlation

Reasoning in CT involves connecting the dots between the pixels and the patient's clinical state. For example, if the agent detects a "ground-glass opacity" in the lungs (Perception), it queries the EHR to check the patient's recent lab results. If the white blood cell count is elevated, it reasons toward "Pneumonia"; if the patient has a history of congestive heart failure, it reasons toward "Pulmonary Edema."

IV. Action: Automated Post-Processing

The CT Agent is an active participant in the workflow. It executes complex "Action" tasks before the radiologist even arrives:

- **Bone Subtraction:** Automatically removing the skull or ribs to better visualize the underlying brain tissue or lungs.
- **Vessel Segmentation:** Tracing the entire path of the aorta to find dissections.
- **3D Reconstruction:** Generating Cinematic Rendering views for surgeons to use in preoperative planning.

High-Impact Use Cases

- **Neurology: The "Stroke Agent"**
  In stroke care, time is brain. The CT Agent acts as an autonomous triage system. Upon completion of a Head CT, the agent immediately analyzes the images for a Large Vessel Occlusion (LVO) or an Intracranial Hemorrhage. If detected, it bypasses all queues and sends

an "urgent alert" to the neuro-interventional team's mobile devices, often cutting the time-to-treatment by 30–60 minutes.

- **Oncology: The "Staging Agent"**
  Cancer staging is one of the most tedious tasks in radiology. A CT Agent can automatically identify and measure lymph nodes across the chest, abdomen, and pelvis. It applies RECIST criteria (Response Evaluation Criteria in Solid Tumors) automatically, comparing current measurements with prior studies to determine if a patient's treatment is working or if the cancer is progressing.

- **Cardiovascular: The "Heart Agent"**
  Modern agents can perform Automated FFR-CT (Fractional Flow Reserve). By simulating blood flow through the 3D model of the coronary arteries, the agent can predict which "clogs" are actually causing a lack of oxygen to the heart, potentially saving the patient from an unnecessary invasive cardiac catheterization.

Workflow Transformation: The "Zero-Click" Paradigm

The ultimate implementation goal in CT is the Zero-Click Workflow. In this model, the radiologist no longer spends time "measuring" or "formatting." Instead, they arrive at their workstation to find a "Draft Report" already populated with 3D measurements, comparisons to previous scans, and a list of key findings. The radiologist's role shifts from "Data Processor" to "Final Decision Maker," allowing them to focus on the clinical nuances that a machine cannot yet grasp.

Building on the volumetric potential of CT, we now look at how the 2026 landscape has integrated AI agents into the very physics of the scanner—optimizing safety, uncovering hidden data, and screening for diseases the patient did not even know they had.

Beyond the Human Eye: Spectral CT and Radiomics

In 2026, the implementation of Spectral (Dual-Energy) CT Agents has revolutionized tissue characterization. Standard CT measures how much an object blocks an X-ray beam, but Spectral CT measures how that blocking changes at different energy levels.

- **Material Decomposition:** The agent can "subtract" calcium to see underlying arterial narrowing or "isolate" iodine to create maps of blood perfusion in the lungs.

- **The "Agentic" Edge:** Manually processing spectral data used to take 10-15 minutes per case. Today's agents perform this decomposition automatically. If the agent detects a pulmonary embolism, it does not just show the clot; it automatically generates a perfused blood volume (PBV) map to show exactly how much lung tissue is being starved of oxygen.

Opportunistic Screening: The "Silent" Guardian

One of the most profound shifts in 21st-century medicine is the move from reactive to proactive care **through Opportunistic** Screening. Every "routine" CT scan contains a wealth of data that goes ignored because it is not relevant to the "Reason for Exam."

- **Hidden Biomarkers:** While a radiologist is focused on a patient's appendix, the Background Agent is busy measuring the bone mineral density of the spine to screen for osteoporosis, calculating the volume of visceral fat to predict metabolic risk, and assessing "sarcopenia" (muscle wasting) to predict surgical outcomes.

- **Case Study:** A patient undergoes a CT for a suspected kidney stone. The agent, running in the background, identifies early-stage coronary artery calcification and vertebral fractures. The agent "reasons" that these are significant and flags them for the primary care physician, potentially preventing a heart attack or hip fracture years down the line.

Radiation Dose Optimization: The AI Shield

The trade-off in CT has always been: "Higher dose = Better image." AI has finally broken this link.

- **Deep Learning Reconstruction (DLR):** Agents now use neural networks to "denoise" images. By understanding what a "perfect" scan should look like, the agent can take a noisy, ultra-low-dose scan and reconstruct it into a diagnostic-quality image.

- **3D Camera Guidance:** In the 2026 suite, the "Physical AI" includes 3D cameras above the gantry. These agents detect the patient's exact body habitus and position, automatically centering them in the "isocenter" of the scanner to ensure the lowest possible radiation exposure while maintaining image clarity.

Limitations: The "Ghost in the Machine"

As we implement these powerful agents, we must remain vigilant against Reconstructive Hallucination. In early iterations of "low-dose" AI, neural networks would occasionally "smooth over" a tiny, real lesion because the algorithm mistook the pathology for image noise. In the high-stakes environment of 2026, "black box" reconstruction is no longer acceptable.

The Digi Health standard for CT agents requires Active Pixel Integrity (API) Check and Residual Mapping.

Instead of simply presenting a "clean" image, the agent maintains a transparent record of its denoising process. If the radiologist is suspicious of an area, they can toggle the Residual Map, which shows exactly what the agent "subtracted" or "altered" from the raw data. This ensures that no subtle, ground-glass opacity or hairline fracture was discarded during the denoising phase. By providing this layer of Pixel-Level Traceability, we bridge the trust gap, ensuring the agent remains a sophisticated advisor that is always subject to human verification.

DIGI HEALTH INSIGHT: The "AI Shield" and the Incidental Save

The Challenge: Balancing Trauma Triage with Fetal Safety A 28-year-old female was admitted to the Emergency Department following a high-velocity motor vehicle accident. The immediate clinical priority was a "Whole-Body Trauma CT" to assess for internal hemorrhaging and spinal fractures. However, the situation was complicated by the patient's clinical history, which revealed she was in her first trimester of pregnancy. This presented a high-risk scenario: the medical team needed life-saving data immediately, but were forced to navigate the extreme radiation sensitivity of a developing fetus.

The Agentic Solution: The Digi Health "Digital Guardian" Operating at the modality edge, the Digi Health CT Agent acted as an autonomous "Digital Guardian" throughout the high-pressure triage.

- **The AI Shield (Precision Dosing):** Before the first photon was emitted, the agent utilized its FHIR-connected interface to verify pregnancy status and body habitus. It autonomously recalibrated the tube current modulation and utilized Deep Learning Reconstruction (DLR). This "AI Shield" achieved a diagnostic-quality scan at a dose 70% lower than standard trauma protocols, ensuring fetal exposure remained well below the safety threshold.

- **Volumetric "Silent Screening":** As the trauma scan was being acquired, the agent's reasoning engine did not sleep. While the human radiologist was clearing the primary trauma (ruling out splenic rupture and aortic dissection), the agent performed a background Geometric Audit of the entire volume.

- **The Critical Catch:** Within seconds of acquisition, the agent flagged a subtle, 4mm suspicious nodule in the patient's thyroid—an area often overlooked during the "tunnel vision" of trauma triage. Using its Longitudinal Memory, it checked the patient's Digital Twin and found no record of thyroid monitoring, identifying this as a high-priority incidental finding.

The Result: From Trauma to Total Care The trauma was cleared, and the patient was stabilized. Because of the AI Shield, the fetal dose was kept within safe margins. More importantly, the agent's "Silent Screening" led to an early-stage diagnosis of thyroid cancer that was entirely unrelated to the accident. The patient was discharged from the ER and directly scheduled for a low-risk endocrine follow-up, transforming a moment of chaos into a life-saving discovery.

Conclusion: From Slices to Solutions

The CT Agent has fundamentally transformed the modality from a passive "slice generator" into a proactive, high-velocity Diagnostic Engine. By mastering the data deluge of the Photon-Counting era, performing autonomous 3D reconstructions, and acting as a Silent Guardian through opportunistic screening, the agent ensures that every photon of radiation delivered to a patient yields the maximum possible clinical value.

In the Digi Health-led department, we have moved beyond the "scroll-and-search" workflows of the early 2000s. The CT suite is no longer a diagnostic bottleneck; it is a high-speed data refinery that feeds the AI Orchestrator with the precise, volumetric truths required for the next stage of care. We are no longer just looking for what we expect to find; we are letting the Agent find what we might otherwise miss.

As we move from the high-energy world of ionizing radiation into the nuanced, magnetic landscapes of the next chapter, the role of the agent shifts from managing volume to managing complexity.

CHAPTER 6: THE PULSE OF LIFE – AI AGENTS IN MRI

Introduction: The Quantum Leap

MRI has always been the gold standard for soft-tissue contrast, yet it remains the primary "bottleneck" of the imaging department. Traditionally, a standard exam requires 30 to 60 minutes of absolute patient stillness. In 2026, the Digi Health MRI Agent has fundamentally rewritten this "quantum" math. We are no longer just "cleaning up" images; we are utilizing autonomous agents to actively steer magnetic gradients, reconstruct data from sparse signals, and manage the patient's biological state in micro-seconds.

The MRI Agent Architecture

MRI requires a significantly more sophisticated reasoning engine than X-ray or CT because the data is acquired in **K-space** (the frequency domain) rather than as direct pixels. To manage this complexity, the agent operates through four integrated layers of intelligence.

I. **Perception: The Signal Guardian**

The MRI agent's perception is divided between the machine and the man.

- **Hardware Perception:** The agent continuously monitors the "health" of the receiver coils and the homogeneity of the magnetic field (shimming), detecting hardware drifts before they result in image artifacts.

- **Patient Perception (The Pulse):** Using Vision-Language Models (VLMs) and non-contact optical sensors, the agent monitors the patient's breathing, heart rate, and even subtle micro-tremors. In 2026, the agent "sees" an irregular breath-hold or a pulse spike and automatically recalibrates the Pulse Sequence in milliseconds to compensate, neutralizing motion blur at the source.

II. **Memory: Multi-Sequence Continuity**

- Unlike other modalities, an MRI exam is a narrative composed of multiple "sequences" (T1, T2, FLAIR, Diffusion). The agent utilizes **Multi-Sequence Memory** to bridge these stages. The agent "remembers" the spatial coordinates of a suspicious lesion detected in the initial T1 sequence and uses that information to optimize the subsequent T2 or Perfusion sequences. If the signal is ambiguous, the agent autonomously "reasons" that it should append a high-resolution 3D sequence to that specific coordinate, ensuring a definitive study without needing a second appointment.

III. Reasoning: The Physics-Informed Reconstruction Engine

- This is the technical core of the 2026 Agentic Shift. Using **Physics-Informed Neural Networks (PINNs)**, the agent reasons about the nature of missing frequency data.

- **Deep Undersampling:** The agent allows the scanner to collect as little as 10% of the standard K-space data, drastically shortening the time the patient spends in the bore.

- **Synthetic Intelligence:** The agent then "reconstructs" the remaining 90% by reasoning through the laws of physics—understanding how water and fat molecules should behave in that specific tissue type. This has transformed the 45-minute lumbar spine scan into a 5-minute **"Flash Scan"** with zero loss in diagnostic fidelity.

IV. Action: The Autonomous Operator

- In the final phase, the agent acts as a **Virtual Technologist**, executing physical changes to the scan environment.

- **Automated Prescription:** The agent identifies anatomical landmarks in real-time to "slice" the heart or brain perfectly every time, regardless of how the patient is positioned.

- **Real-time Correction:** If a patient moves significantly, the agent's primary "Action" is to pause the sequence, calculate the new spatial coordinates, and restart the specific scan segment without human intervention, ensuring every exam is "Right the First Time."

High-Impact Use Cases

- **Neurology: The "Neuro-Degenerative Watchman"**
  - In 2026, agents like NextBrain use high-resolution "Brain Atlases" to monitor aging.
  - **Volumetric Analysis:** The agent automatically segments 300+ brain regions, measuring the volume of the hippocampus and amygdala.

- **Trend Reasoning:** It compares these volumes to a database of thousands of patients to flag early signs of Alzheimer's or Parkinson's years before clinical symptoms appear.

- **Cardiovascular: The "Living Heart"**
  MRI of the heart is notoriously difficult because the heart is always moving. Cardiac AI Agents now perform "Real-time Cine" imaging. They can track the heart's wall motion and calculate the "Ejection Fraction" (how much blood the heart pumps) in real-time, providing immediate feedback on cardiac health during the scan.

- **Oncology: The "Virtual Biopsy"**
  Through Radiomics, the MRI agent analyzes the "texture" of a tumor. In prostate or breast imaging, the agent can predict if a lesion is malignant or benign with 95% accuracy by analyzing the diffusion of water molecules, often reducing the need for painful physical biopsies.

Workflow Integration: The 15-Minute Full Body Scan

The ultimate implementation milestone of 2026 is the $500, 15-minute full-body MRI. By combining accelerated reconstruction with autonomous "Scout" agents that navigate from head to toe, MRI is transitioning from a "problem-solving" tool for sick patients to a "screening" tool for healthy ones.

In 2026, the MRI suite has been transformed by agents that go beyond mere image processing; they are now actively synthesizing data that was never physically recorded, effectively "filling in the blanks" of human biology.

Beyond the Needle: Synthetic Contrast

One of the most significant breakthroughs in the 2026 landscape is Synthetic Contrast. Traditionally, highlighting tumors required the injection of Gadolinium-based contrast agents (GBCAs).

- **The Virtual Agent:** Utilizing a Generative Adversarial Network (GAN), the MRI Agent reasons what a contrast-enhanced scan *would* look like based on high-resolution non-contrast data.

- **Clinical Impact:** While real contrast remains the gold standard for surgery, "Virtual Gadolinium" has reduced diagnostic needle sticks by 40%, particularly in pediatric and chronic-care populations where venous access is difficult.

The "Motionless" Patient: Dynamic Real-Time Correction

Motion has historically been the "Achilles' heel" of MRI. A single sneeze or a slight shift in position by a claustrophobic patient could ruin a 20-minute sequence, requiring a complete restart.

- **The Vision-Loop Correction:** In 2026, the MRI gantry is equipped with integrated high-speed optical cameras that track the patient's skin and eyes at 60 frames per second.

- **Agentic Compensation:** This "Perception" data is fed directly into the magnetic gradient controller. If the patient moves their head 2mm to the left, the agent "reasons" the necessary coordinate shift and "acts" by adjusting the magnetic field in real-time. To the radiologist, the patient appears to have been perfectly still, as the "virtual camera" of the MRI followed the movement exactly.

Pediatric MRI: Sedation-Free Scans

The combination of high-speed reconstruction and motion correction has had its most profound impact on pediatric imaging.

- **The End of Anesthesia:** Traditionally, children often required general anesthesia just to remain still for an MRI—a process with inherent neurological risks.

- **The "Swift" Protocol:** By utilizing "Agentic Stealth" (sequences that are quieter) and "Flash Reconstruction" (sequences that take seconds rather than minutes), hospitals in 2026 are achieving a "90% Sedation-Free" rate for pediatric neuro-imaging. The agent acts as a guardian, monitoring the child's comfort and adjusting the scan speed dynamically.

Technical Implementation: The Computational Challenge

The technical burden of an MRI agent is significantly higher than that of X-ray or CT.

- **K-Space Pipelines:** Because MRI data is frequency-based, the agent must perform "Fast Fourier Transforms" (FFT) in parallel with its neural network inferences. This requires massive on-site GPU clusters or dedicated fiber-optic links to "Regional AI Hubs."

- **Bio-Security and Privacy:** Since MRI images are so detailed they can technically be "re-identified" (by reconstructing the patient's face from a brain scan), the agent includes an automated **"Defacing" module**. Before any data leaves the local secure environment for cloud-based "Memory" retrieval, the agent autonomously strips away non-diagnostic identifiable features.

Limitations: The "Smoothness" Bias

While MRI agents are remarkably good at denoising and accelerating scans, they can occasionally suffer from "Over-Smoothing." If the agent's "Reasoning" is too aggressive, it might mistake a very fine, subtle tear in a ligament for "noise" and smooth it out. In 2026, we mitigate this with **Uncertainty Maps**. If the agent is unsure about a specific pixel cluster, it leaves it "raw," signaling to the radiologist: "I couldn't confidently reconstruct this area; please pay close attention."

DIGI HEALTH INSIGHT: The "Seven-Minute" Neuro-Oncology Protocol

The Challenge: The Motion-Intolerance Bottleneck In late 2024, a 45-year-old patient presented with a suspected recurrence of a glioblastoma (GBM). Standard neuro-oncology MRI protocols are notoriously grueling, typically requiring 45 to 60 minutes of absolute immobility across multiple sequences. The patient, suffering from post-surgical claustrophobia and mild cognitive impairment, was unable to remain still. Traditional imaging attempts resulted in severe motion artifacts, rendering the scans non-diagnostic and leaving the surgical team without a clear path forward.

The Agentic Solution: The Digi Health "Autonomous Session" To salvage the diagnostic window, the department deployed the Digi Health MRI Agent to take over the session and steer the scanner in real-time.

- **Physics-Informed "Flash" Reconstruction:** Rather than attempting a traditional full-data acquisition, the agent utilized Physics-Informed Neural Networks (PINNs) to perform a deep-undersampled scan. By collecting only 15% of the standard K-space frequencies, the agent "reasoned" the remaining 85% based on the patient's biological tissue signatures, maintaining diagnostic SNR (Signal-to-Noise Ratio) while slashing acquisition time.

- **Autonomous Protocol Steering:** Within the first 120 seconds, the agent's reasoning engine detected a subtle, ambiguous signal enhancement near the surgical bed. Utilizing its Multi-Sequence Memory, the agent autonomously "pushed" an unscheduled, high-resolution 3D-Perfusion sequence to that specific coordinate. It realized that differentiating between radiation necrosis and true tumor recurrence was the "true" clinical question, and it secured that data without human prompting.

- **Vision-Loop Guarding:** When the patient's breathing became erratic due to anxiety, the VLM (Vision-Language Model) sensors detected the chest wall excursion. The agent adjusted the magnetic gradients at 60Hz to compensate for the physical movement, "locking" the image in place despite the patient's restlessness.

The Result: From Agitation to Actionable Intelligence A comprehensive, diagnostic-quality neuro-oncology exam—which would normally take an hour—was completed in exactly 7 minutes and 12 seconds. The agent immediately drafted a structured preliminary report and "pushed" the findings to the neurosurgeon's device via a secure FHIR-based alert. By the time the patient was being helped out of the scanner, the surgical team was already reviewing the updated tumor maps to plan the next intervention.

Conclusion: Capturing the Pulse of Life

The MRI Agent has achieved what was once considered a physical impossibility: it has taken the most complex diagnostic tool in medicine and made it fast, safe, and truly accessible. By bridging the gap between quantum frequency domains and real-time clinical reality, these agents have transformed the "bottleneck" of the hospital into its most powerful engine of discovery.

We have moved beyond an era where patients had to endure hour-long sessions in a magnetic bore. In the Digi Health-enabled suite, the Pulse of Life is captured in minutes, with "Synthetic Contrast" reducing the need for invasive needles and "Vision-Loop" corrections eliminating the risk of motion-blurred data. These agents do not just reconstruct images; they reconstruct the patient experience.

As we conclude our look at the "Big Three" modalities—X-ray, CT, and MRI—we turn our attention to the most personal and portable tool in the clinician's arsenal. In the next chapter, we will see how Agentic AI is transforming the "hand-held" world of Ultrasound, bringing world-class diagnostic vision to the point of care.

CHAPTER 7: THE SOUND OF SIGHT – AI AGENTS IN ULTRASOUND

Introduction: Breaking the "Skill Barrier"

Ultrasound is unique because it is "dynamic." Unlike a CT scan, which follows a pre-set mechanical path, ultrasound images are created in real-time by the human operator's hand. If the probe is tilted one millimeter too far, a life-threatening gallstone or fetal abnormality can simply vanish from the screen. This "operator dependence" has traditionally restricted ultrasound to highly trained specialists.

The Digi Health Ultrasound Agent acts as a "GPS for the Human Body." It does not just analyze the image after it is captured; it guides the hand while it is moving. This shift has enabled Point-of-Care Ultrasound (POCUS) to become a universal vital sign, effectively replacing the stethoscope as the primary tool of physical examination.

The Ultrasound Agent Architecture: Real-Time Guidance

Because ultrasound is a "live" modality, the agentic loop (Perception-Reasoning-Action) must operate at a staggering 60 frames per second.

I. **Perception: The Spatial Navigator**

The agent's perception is "dual-track."

- **External Perception:** Many 2026 handheld probes include integrated cameras or inertial sensors that track the probe's position in 3D space relative to the patient's body.
- **Internal Perception:** The agent analyzes the live video stream, identifying anatomical "landmarks" (like the spine or the aorta) to understand exactly where the beam is hitting.

II. **Memory: The "Ideal" Template**

Ultrasound agents utilize Atlas-Based Memory. The agent has "memorized" millions of perfect scans across all body types. As you move the probe, the agent compares your live, "messy" view to its internal "ideal" template. It "remembers" what the four chambers of the heart *should* look like from your current angle and identifies the "gap" between your image and a diagnostic-quality one.

III. Reasoning: The Guiding Logic

Active Feedback Coaching The reasoning engine acts as a live coach. Using Active Feedback Reasoning, the agent provides haptic or visual instructions: *"Tilt 5° cephalad"* or *"Increase compression to displace bowel gas."* This transforms a novice user into an expert-level scanner in a single session.

IV. Action: Automated Quantification

In ultrasound, "Action" is about removing the manual labor of measurement.

- **Auto-Labeling:** The agent automatically identifies and labels the liver, kidneys, and spleen in real-time.

- **Auto-EF (Ejection Fraction):** In cardiac imaging, the agent "acts" by automatically tracing the heart's borders as it beats, calculating the heart's strength instantly without the doctor needing to "freeze" and draw lines manually.

- **Robotic Navigation:** In advanced 2026 surgical suites, AI agents drive Robotic Ultrasound Arms, performing completely autonomous scans of the carotid arteries or the thyroid with zero human contact.

High-Impact Use Cases

- **Obstetrics: The "Safe-Start" Agent**

In maternal health, agents are used to identify standard fetal planes automatically. For a rural midwife, the agent can confirm the baby's position, measure the head circumference, and estimate the amniotic fluid volume with a single sweep of the probe. If the agent detects a potential anomaly, it automatically uploads the clip to a specialist for review.

- **Emergency Medicine: The "Crash" Agent**

During a trauma resuscitation, a "FAST" (Focused Assessment with Sonography for Trauma) exam is critical. The Ultrasound Agent can identify internal bleeding in the abdomen within seconds, even in a chaotic, moving environment. It provides a simple "Green/Red" indicator for "Free Fluid Detected," allowing the trauma team to move straight to surgery.

- **Vascular: The "Deep Vein" Guardian**

Detecting blood clots (DVT) in the legs is a high-volume task. 2026 agents use Compression Logic. The agent monitors the probe pressure and observes if the vein "collapses." If the vein remains open under pressure, the agent flags a potential clot and automatically generates a vascular map for the clinician.

Workflow Transformation: The "Democratized" Clinic

The true power of the Ultrasound Agent is its ability to move the diagnostic room to the patient's bedside. By 2026, handheld ultrasound devices are as common as smartphones. Because the agent ensures "Diagnostic-Level Quality" regardless of the user's experience, we are seeing:

- **Nurse-Led Screening:** Nurses performing routine heart and lung checks during rounds.
- **Home-Based Monitoring:** Patients with chronic heart failure using "Agent-Guided" home probes to check for fluid buildup in their lungs, preventing hospital readmissions.

In 2026, the transition of ultrasound from a "specialist-only" tool to a universal medical "vital sign" is being driven by a profound shift in hardware. We are no longer just looking at miniaturized versions of big machines; we are witnessing the era of Ultrasound-on-Chip technology.

Ultrasound-on-Chip: The AI Inside the Transducer

The most radical technical shift in 2026 is the replacement of traditional piezoelectric crystals with Capacitive Micromachined Ultrasonic Transducers (CMUT) and photonics-based chips.

- **On-Chip Intelligence:** Traditionally, ultrasound data had to be sent from the probe to a bulky console for processing. In 2026, the AI agent lives directly on the silicon chip within the handheld probe. This "Intelligence at the Source" allows for Digital Beamforming, where the agent optimizes the acoustic wave thousands of times per second based on the tissue it is hitting.

- **Cell-Phone Integration:** Because the processing happens on-chip, these probes can plug directly into a standard smartphone. The agent uses the phone's GPU to render the final image, making "Diagnostic-Grade" imaging available for the price of a high-end consumer gadget.

Tele-Ultrasound: The "Ghost" in the Hand

In rural or low-resource settings, the Ultrasound Agent acts as a bridge to specialized care through **Collaborative Tele-Ultrasound**.

- **The "Driver-Assist" Model:** A nurse in a remote clinic can hold the probe while a specialist hundreds of miles away sees the live stream. However, unlike old-fashioned video calls, the Tele-Agent handles the quality control.

- **Automated Sufficiency:** If the signal is too weak or the probe is in the wrong place, the agent pauses the stream and provides the nurse with 3D graphical overlays to correct the position. The specialist only receives a "notification" once the agent confirms the image is of diagnostic quality. This "One-to-Many" model allows a single radiologist to supervise dozens of bedside exams simultaneously.

Continuous Monitoring: The Ultrasound Patch

The ultimate evolution of the ultrasound agent in 2026 is the move from *episodic* scans to *continuous* monitoring.

- **The Wearable Patch:** New "Smart Patches" can be adhered to a patient's chest or neck. These contain miniature ultrasound arrays managed by a low-power AI agent.

- **Home-Based Triage:** For patients with chronic heart failure, the patch monitors the lungs for early signs of fluid (pulmonary edema). If the agent detects a "trend" toward congestion—even before the patient feels short of breath—it "acts" by alerting the remote care team. This shifts ultrasound from a "test" you go to the hospital for, into a "monitor" that lives with you.

Limitations: The "Over-Confidence" Trap

As ultrasound becomes more accessible, the primary risk in 2026 is unskilled over-reliance. If a non-expert user sees a "Green Light" from the agent indicating a "Normal" scan, they may stop looking for rare anomalies the agent was not trained to see.

- **Human-in-the-Loop Safeguards:** To combat this, 2026 agents are required to show **"Certainty Maps."** If an agent identifies a structure but has a low confidence score, it will force the user to capture "secondary views" to confirm the finding, ensuring that the machine's speed never compromises clinical safety.

DIGI HEALTH INSIGHT: The "Autonomous Sonographer"

The Challenge: The Rural Cardiac Gap A rural clinic lacked a specialized cardiac sonographer. A patient presented with acute shortness of breath. The general technologist on-site struggled to capture the "Gold Standard" apical four-chamber view required to rule out heart failure.

The Agentic Solution: The Digi Health Live Guide

- **Real-Time Navigation:** Through the tablet interface, the agent provided visual cues (arrows and tilt-degree indicators) to help the technologist find the optimal acoustic window through the ribs.

- **Auto-Capture & Reasoning:** Once the agent recognized the "Ideal" view, it autonomously "froze" the frame and performed a Biplane calculation for Ejection Fraction.

The Result: A diagnostic-quality echo was performed by a generalist. Congestive heart failure was diagnosed on the spot, allowing for immediate treatment without a 100-mile transfer to a city hospital.

Conclusion: The Democratization of Vision

By moving intelligence directly onto the chip and providing real-time "GPS" guidance, the Ultrasound Agent has democratized medical imaging. It has taken a modality that traditionally required years of intensive "hand-eye" mastery and turned it into a high-fidelity tool that any clinician—and in some cases, even a patient at home—can use to monitor health and save lives.

However, as we move from the portable, hand-held world of ultrasound, we encounter a different set of challenges: the sub-atomic world of molecular imaging. In the next chapter, we move to PET and Nuclear Medicine, where AI agents stop guiding the human hand and start mastering the physics of individual photons to visualize the very chemistry of disease.

CHAPTER 8: THE MOLECULAR VIEW – AI AGENTS IN PET AND NUCLEAR MEDICINE

In this chapter, we move from the anatomical and functional views of CT and MRI to the molecular frontier of Nuclear Medicine. While other modalities show us what the body *looks like*, PET (Positron Emission Tomography) and SPECT (Single-Photon Emission Computed Tomography) show us how the body *is behaving* at a cellular level. In 2026, Molecular AI Agents have turned Nuclear Medicine from a slow, "grainy" specialty into a high-precision tool for "Theranostics"—the integration of therapy and diagnostics.

Introduction: Visualizing the Invisible

Nuclear medicine is the "biology" of imaging. By injecting radioactive tracers that target specific metabolic pathways, we can see cancer cells consuming glucose or detect the first signs of Alzheimer's amyloid plaques. However, PET and SPECT have historically been limited by two factors: high radiation doses and "noisy," grainy images that require long acquisition times.

The Digi Health Molecular Agent of 2026 has fundamentally altered this equation. By applying the "Perception-Reasoning-Action" loop to the photon level, these agents allow us to see deeper into the human cell than ever before, using a fraction of the traditional radioactive dose.

The Nuclear Agent Architecture: The Photon Master

Because Nuclear Medicine involves detecting individual gamma rays or positrons, the agent operates at the sub-millisecond level of List-Mode Data.

I. **Perception: The Scintillation Guardian**

The agent's perception begins at the detector crystal.

- **Ultra-Low-Count Perception:** In 2026, Digi Health agents are trained to perceive patterns in "sparse data." This allows for a 50–80% reduction in injected radioactive tracers. The agent "sees" the rare photons and uses deep learning to distinguish between "true signal" (the tumor) and "background noise" (natural radiation).

- **4D Motion Binning:** PET scans are notoriously sensitive to breathing. The agent perceives the patient's respiratory cycle in real-time and "bins" photons into the correct phase of the breath, creating a 4D image that remains perfectly sharp even in the moving lungs.

II. Memory: Pharmacokinetic Tracking

Molecular agents utilize Pharmacokinetic Memory. The agent "remembers" the specific metabolic signature of tracers like FDG (glucose) or PSMA (prostate-specific membrane antigen). It compares the "uptake" at 10 minutes versus 60 minutes, reasoning about the metabolic "velocity" of a tumor to determine if it is aggressive or responding to therapy.

III. Reasoning: The Theranostic Bridge

This is the "Brain" of the 2026 Nuclear Agent, where diagnostics (seeing) meets therapy (treating).

- **Dosimetry Reasoning:** If a patient is receiving radioactive therapy (like Lutetium-177), the agent calculates exactly how much radiation is hitting the tumor versus sensitive healthy organs like the kidneys. It calculates the Personalized Absorbed Dose in real-time, maximizing the "kill rate" for cancer while minimizing side effects.

IV. Action: The Automated Molecular Quantifier

" Action" here is the elimination of human subjectivity in measuring metabolic activity.

- **Auto-SUV Orchestration:** The agent "acts" by automatically identifying every "hot spot" in the body, calculating its volume and Standardized Uptake Value (SUV). It then compares these to a global database via MCP to categorize them as "Likely Malignant" or "Post-Inflammatory.

High-Impact Use Cases

- **Oncology: Total-Body PET Agents**
  In 2026, "Long-Axis" PET scanners can image the whole body at once. A Whole-Body Agent can track a cancer's "metabolic footprint" from head to toe in under 60 seconds. It identifies "micro-metastases" (tiny cancer spread) that would be invisible on a standard scan, allowing for truly "Precision Oncology."

- **Neurology: The Amyloid Watchman**
  For dementia, PET agents analyze the density of amyloid and tau proteins in the brain. The agent does not just provide a "Yes/No" for Alzheimer's; it provides a "Prognostic Reasoning," predicting the likely rate of cognitive decline over the next 24 months based on the molecular pattern.

- **Cardiology: The Ischemia Agent**
  In cardiac SPECT, agents analyze blood flow to the heart muscle. The agent "acts" by automatically generating a "Risk Map," identifying which specific coronary artery needs a stent based on the molecular stress test, reducing the time from scan to surgery.

Workflow Transformation: The "Dose-on-Demand" Suite

The ultimate implementation of 2026 is the Ultra-Low Dose PET. Because the agent is so good at "denoising," we have moved PET from a "high-radiation" last resort to a tool that can be used for routine screening and frequent treatment monitoring.

In 2026, the molecular precision of Nuclear Medicine is no longer a slow, grainy endeavor. By leveraging high-dimensional data and synthetic processing, AI agents are pushing the boundaries of what can be detected—and treated—at the photon level.

Synthetic PET-CT Fusion: The "Unified" Vision

Traditionally, hybrid imaging like PET-CT required a patient to undergo two separate scans, with the computer later "stitching" them together. In 2026, the AI agent performs Deep-Fused Synthesis.

- **Anatomical Hallucination Prevention:** One of the historic risks of AI was "hallucinating" anatomy. The 2026 agent uses Cross-Modality Transformers to ensure that the metabolic "hot spot" (PET) perfectly aligns with the anatomical structure (CT). If the patient moves between the two acquisitions, the agent performs a voxel-level "warp" in real-time to maintain 100% spatial registration.

- **Virtual CT Attenuation:** In cases where a CT scan cannot be performed (due to contrast allergies or radiation concerns), advanced agents can synthesize a "Virtual CT" from the PET emission data alone. This provides the necessary "map" for attenuation correction without the extra radiation of a secondary X-ray source.

Beyond the Image: Radiomics and the "Digital Biopsy"

While a radiologist looks at the "brightness" of a tumor (SUV), the Radiomics Agent looks at the Texture.

- **The Invisible Signature:** The agent extracts thousands of high-dimensional features—such as entropy, skewness, and voxel heterogeneity—that are invisible to the human eye.

- **Tumor Phenotyping:** By analyzing these patterns, the agent can reason about the "Tumor Microenvironment." It can predict if a lung cancer has a specific genetic mutation (e.g., EGFR or KRAS) just by looking at the metabolic "noise" within the PET pixels. This "Digital Biopsy" allows for targeted therapy to begin days before the physical pathology results return from the lab.

Radiation Safety: The "ALARA" AI

The fundamental principle of Nuclear Medicine is ALARA (As Low As Reasonably Achievable). In 2026, AI agents are the primary enforcement mechanism for this goal.

- **Low-Dose Reconstruction (DLR):** Through Deep Learning-based Reconstruction, 2026 agents can produce diagnostic-quality images using only 1% to 10% of the standard radioactive tracer dose. This is particularly vital in pediatric oncology, where the cumulative lifetime radiation dose is a major concern.
- **Automated Dosimetry:** For patients undergoing radiopharmaceutical therapy (Theranostics), the agent acts as a "Safety Monitor." It tracks the tracer's residence time in sensitive organs like the kidneys and bone marrow. If the agent reasons that the "absorbed dose" is approaching a toxic threshold, it automatically triggers a "Dose Adjustment" recommendation for the next cycle.

Technical Implementation: The Computational Heavyweight

Handling photon-level data requires immense processing power.

- **GPU Pipelines:** PET agents in 2026 utilize massive parallelization. The "List-Mode" data (the raw timestamps of every detected photon) is processed through GPU-accelerated neural networks to reconstruct the 3D volume in under 60 seconds.
- **DICOM-RT Integration:** For therapy planning, the agent utilizes DICOM-RT (Radiotherapy) standards to export its molecular maps directly into the treatment planning systems, ensuring the "Digital Colleague" is integrated across the entire oncology department.

DIGI HEALTH INSIGHT: The "Molecular Time Machine"

The Challenge: A PET/CT scan for oncology staging often suffers from "Image Noise" due to short tracer half-lives or low-dose protocols intended to protect the patient.

The Agentic Solution: Cross-Modality Fusion The Digi Health Molecular Agent utilized Anatomical Hallucination Prevention to solve this.

- **Structural Priors:** The agent used the high-resolution CT "Digital Twin" as an anatomical map to "denoise" the PET signal without losing metabolic sensitivity.

- **Predictive Uptake:** It identified a faint "hot spot" that was below the standard SUV (Standardized Uptake Value) threshold but, based on the LMM's knowledge of this specific cancer subtype, identified it as an early-stage metastasis.

The Result: The agent transformed a low-dose, "noisy" scan into a high-definition metabolic map. It caught the spread of disease months earlier than traditional software, allowing the patient to start advanced systemic therapy immediately and avoiding a "false negative" that could have been fatal.

Conclusion: From Grainy to Genetic

The Molecular Agent has achieved a feat once thought impossible: it has transformed Nuclear Medicine from a noisy, "blurry" science into a high-fidelity tool of genetic and metabolic precision. By navigating the sub-millisecond world of photon-level data, these agents have moved beyond simply "taking a picture" to performing a real-time Biochemical Audit of the human body.

By synthesizing data across modalities and extracting "invisible" textures through Radiomics, the Digi Health Molecular Agent has made the hidden processes of cellular life perfectly clear. We no longer wait for a tumor to grow large enough to be seen; we detect it while it is still a metabolic whisper.

We have now traveled from the structural "workhorse" of X-ray to the molecular frontier of PET. However, the true test of an agent is its ability to find the "needle in the haystack" during high-stakes screening. In the next chapter, we move into the specialized world of Mammography, where AI agents are solving the crisis of "density" and ensuring that early detection is a reality for every patient.

CHAPTER 9: THE SPECIALIZED EYE – AI AGENTS IN MAMMOGRAPHY

In this chapter, we address the unique complexities of women's health. In our 2026 "Digi Health" vision, Mammography has evolved from a simple screening tool into a Predictive Health Engine. The AI Agent is no longer just a "second set of eyes"—it is a navigator through the "fog" of dense breast tissue.

Introduction: The High-Stakes Search

Breast cancer screening is a high-volume, high-consequence field. A radiologist may look at 100 mammograms in a single session, knowing that only a small fraction will contain a malignancy. The challenge is two-fold: Perception (finding the tiny cluster of calcifications) and Masking (finding cancer hidden behind dense breast tissue).

In 2026, the Digi Health Mammography Agent has moved beyond simple "box-drawing" CAD tools. We now utilize agents that can predict cancer risk five years before a tumor appears, transforming mammography from a retrospective search into a proactive diagnostic pathway.

The Mammography Agent Architecture

The architecture for women's health must be exceptionally precise to handle the subtle symmetries of breast tissue.

I. **Perception: The Symmetry Analyst**

The agent's perception is built on Bilateral and Temporal Comparison.

- **Comparing Left to Right:** The agent simultaneously analyzes the left and right breasts. It "perceives" asymmetries that are often the first sign of a developing tumor, even when no discrete mass is visible.
- **3D Tomosynthesis Integration:** In 2026, Digital Breast Tomosynthesis (DBT) is the standard. The agent "sees" through the 1-mm slices of the breast volume, identifying "Architectural Distortion"—a subtle pulling of tissue—that often precedes a visible lump.

II. Memory: The Five-Year Vision

One of the greatest breakthroughs of 2026 is Predictive Longitudinal Memory.

- **Longitudinal Patterning:** The agent does not just look at the last two years of scans; it analyzes the patient's entire imaging history.

- **The Five-Year Risk Score:** By recognizing "pre-cancerous" patterns in the texture of the breast—patterns invisible to the human eye—the agent can assign a personalized 5-year risk score. This allows high-risk women to be moved into more intensive screening (like MRI) before a tumor ever forms.

III. Reasoning: The Density Navigator

Breast density is a major hurdle in mammography; dense tissue appears white on a scan, the same color as cancer.

- **Automated Density Stratification:** The agent "reasons" the exact volumetric density of the breast (BI-RADS A-D).

- **Supplemental Pathfinding:** If a patient has "Extremely Dense" breasts (Category D), the agent automatically reasons that the mammogram is "Incomplete" and triggers an **Action** to recommend a follow-up automated ultrasound or MRI.

IV. Action: The Worklist Prioritizer

The agent acts as a "Safety Net" in the screening workflow.

- **Smart Prioritization:** The agent scans the day's mammograms in the background. If it finds a "High-Confidence Malignancy" (BI-RADS 5), it moves that patient to the very top of the radiologist's worklist, often allowing for a same-day biopsy.

- **Drafting the Report:** The agent automatically populates the density score, the location of findings, and the comparison to prior years, reducing the radiologist's typing time by 40%.

Key Clinical Use Cases

- **The "Interval Cancer" Shield**

"Interval cancers" are those that appear in the 12–24 months between regular screenings. In 2026, AI agents are used to re-analyze "Normal" mammograms from the previous year. Studies have shown that AI can "back-detect" subtle signs of interval cancers in up to 76% of cases, allowing clinicians to catch these aggressive tumors much earlier.

- **Precision Screening**

Not every woman needs a mammogram every year; some need more, some need less.

Personalized Pathways: Based on the agent's 5-year risk score, women in 2026 receive personalized screening schedules. A woman with low density and a "Low AI Risk Score" may move to biennial screening, while a woman with high density and a "High AI Risk Score" is fast-tracked for specialized 3D imaging.

- **Technical Implementation: Explainable AI**

In mammography, trust is paramount.

- **Saliency Maps:** The 2026 agent does not just say "Cancer found." It provides a "Heatmap" or "Saliency Map" that shows exactly which pixels triggered the alert.

- **Feature Justification:** The agent provides a list of "Reasons," such as *"Spiculated margin detected"* or *"Pleomorphic calcifications present,"* allowing the radiologist to verify the machine's logic instantly.

DIGI HEALTH INSIGHT: The "Clinical Sentinel"

The Challenge: The Density Dilemma. A 52-year-old patient with dense breast tissue (Category C) underwent her annual 3D Tomosynthesis. Traditional CAD (Computer-Aided Detection) software often struggles with dense tissue, leading to high false-positive rates that cause unnecessary patient anxiety or, conversely, "masking" that hides early-stage malignancies.

The Agentic Solution: The Digi Health Mammography Agent acted as a Clinical Sentinel, moving beyond mere pixel-pattern recognition.

- **Longitudinal Reasoning:** The agent did not just look at the current scan. It autonomously retrieved the patient's prior mammograms from the last five years, using Deformable Registration to track the exact "evolution" of tissue density at the micron level.

- **Multimodal Correlation (MCP):** Simultaneously, the agent queried the EHR for the patient's latest Genomic Risk Score and hormone replacement therapy history. It "reasoned" that a specific, subtle architectural distortion—which might have been dismissed as a scar—was actually high-risk given her genetic profile.

- **Autonomous Escalation:** Before the radiologist even opened the case, the agent had already flagged the specific slice in the 3D volume and pre-scheduled a follow-up Automated Breast Ultrasound (ABUS) for the same afternoon, ensuring no time was lost in the diagnostic pathway.

The Result: The Single-Visit Diagnosis. A small, 6mm invasive ductal carcinoma was detected in a "masking" area of dense tissue. By integrating longitudinal history with genetic data, the agent provided a "Single-Visit Diagnosis," eliminating the standard 14-day wait for follow-up results and significantly improving the patient's prognosis.

Conclusion: From Volume to Victory

By integrating longitudinal history with real-time multimodal reasoning, the Mammography Agent has fundamentally transformed breast imaging from a reactive "search for disease" into a proactive Predictive Health Engine. It effectively bridges the gap between the static pixel and the complex patient narrative, solving the "Masking" challenge of dense tissue while simultaneously providing a digital safety net for the detection of aggressive "Interval Cancers."

In the agentic era, mammography is no longer just a high-stakes volume game; it is a personalized diagnostic pathway. Here, the machine provides the Calculation—the tireless, micron-level analysis of symmetry and texture—so that the physician can provide the final Judgment and Compassion. This partnership ensures that in the most sensitive of clinical moments, no finding is lost to density, and no patient is lost to the system.

CHAPTER 10: THE PRECISION CO-PILOT – AI AGENTS IN INTERVENTIONAL RADIOLOGY

In 2026, the interventional radiology (IR) suite is no longer a place of "guesswork and grit." It has evolved into a high-tech cockpit where the radiologist acts as a mission commander, supported by an AI agent that serves as both a navigator and a precision engineer.

Introduction: From Static to Dynamic

Traditional radiology is a retrospective science—it deals with the "Past" (the scan captured an hour ago). Interventional Radiology (IR) is about the Now. In the IR suite, clinicians perform surgery through pinholes, navigating catheters through miles of microscopic vessels to deliver life-saving treatments.

Historically, this required extreme mental gymnastics—mentally mapping a static 3D CT scan onto a live, flickering 2D X-ray (fluoroscopy) screen. The Digi Health IR Agent of 2026 eliminates this cognitive load. It does not just show the doctor where the catheter is; it serves as a high-tech "cockpit" that shows them where it *should* be, providing a digital safety net that prevents complications before they occur.

The IR Agent Architecture: The Surgical Loop

Because IR is a live "contact sport," the agentic architecture must be faster and more tactile than in any other modality.

I. Perception: Multimodal Fusion & Real-Time Tracking

The IR Agent's perception is built on **Hyper-Fusion**.

- **3D-to-2D Overlay:** The agent takes the high-resolution "road map" from the patient's pre-operative CT or MRI and "pins" it to the live fluoroscopy video. If the patient breathes or the table moves, the agent's Motion-Tracking Perception adjusts the 3D map in milliseconds, ensuring the "digital road" always aligns with the "physical vessel."

- **Instrument Recognition:** Using computer vision, the agent identifies the specific tip of the needle or catheter. It "perceives" the distance between the needle and a critical structure (like an artery wall) and provides haptic or visual warnings if the surgeon gets too close.

II. **Memory: Case-Specific Patterning** The agent utilizes Procedural Memory to guide the surgeon's hand

- **Global Patterning:** The agent utilizes Case-Specific Memory. It queries the global database for thousands of similar procedures (e.g., "difficult splenic artery embolization"). If it "remembers" that 90% of similar cases failed using a certain catheter angle, it flags this to the surgeon *before* they make the turn.

- **Intra-Procedural Context:** The agent maintains a "State Log" of the current surgery. It remembers every milliliter of contrast injected and every second of radiation used, alerting the team if the patient is approaching safety thresholds.

III. **Reasoning: The Predictive Navigator**

In 2026, we utilize Physics-Informed Reasoning to predict outcomes before they happen.

- **Ablation Zone Prediction:** During tumor ablation (killing cancer with heat or cold), the agent "reasons" the outcome. It analyzes the local blood flow (which acts as a "heat sink") and predicts exactly how large the "kill zone" will be. If the predicted zone does not cover the entire tumor, the agent suggests a new needle position.

- **Vascular Pathfinder:** For stroke or aneurysm cases, the agent calculates the "Path of Least Resistance." It reasons through the vessel tortuosity to suggest the optimal sequence of wires to reach the target faster, saving precious brain tissue.

IV. **Action: Robotic Control & Touchless Orchestration**

The "Action" phase in IR is about physical precision.

- **Robotic Assistance:** The agent "acts" by driving Micro-Robotic Steerable **Catheters**. The surgeon provides the high-level intent ("Go to the left hepatic artery"), and the agent executes the sub-millimeter movements required to get there, eliminating the "hand tremors" that can occur during long, stressful procedures.

- **The "Zero-Touch" Interface:** To maintain a sterile environment, the agent responds to Voice and Gesture Control. A surgeon can say, *"Agent, show me the 2024 PET scan overlay,"* or wave their hand to rotate a 3D model of the patient's heart, without ever touching a mouse or keyboard.

High-Impact Use Cases: The Stroke and Cancer Frontiers

- **Neurology: The "Thrombectomy Co-Pilot"**
  In mechanical thrombectomy (removing a clot from the brain), every minute counts. The IR Agent identifies the "Clot Architecture" and suggests the exact size of the stent-riever needed. It guides the catheter with such precision that "re-canalization" (restoring blood flow) happens in one pass instead of three, drastically improving patient recovery rates.

- **Oncology: The "Precision Ablator"**
  For liver or kidney tumors, the agent acts as an architect. It uses Radiomics to see the "micro-margins" of the tumor. By providing a 3D visual of the "safety buffer," it ensures the surgeon kills the cancer without damaging the adjacent healthy tissue or major blood vessels.

Workflow Transformation: The "Invisible" Safe Suite

The ultimate goal of implementation is the Radiation-Silent Procedure.

- **Synthetic Fluoro:** By using AI to "guess" the frames between X-ray pulses, the agent allows the surgeon to operate with a "smooth" video at an ultra-low pulse rate. This has reduced the radiation dose for IR staff and patients by up to 70% in 2026.
- **Automated Coding and Notes:** As the procedure ends, the agent "acts" by generating a complete operative report. It lists every device used, the total contrast volume, and the final result, allowing the surgeon to move to the next patient immediately.

To illustrate the power of agentic AI in the surgical suite, let us look at a "Day in the Life" case study from a leading Comprehensive Stroke Center in 2026. This scenario demonstrates how the AI Agent moves from Perception to Action to save a patient's life during the "Golden Hour."

Case Study: The "Shadow Surgeon" – A 2026 Stroke Thrombectomy

The Patient: Elena, 68, arrives at a rural community hospital with sudden right-sided paralysis and loss of speech.

1. Pre-Procedural Triage (The Handoff)

- **The Agent's Perception:** As soon as Elena's initial Head CT is completed at the local hospital, the **Neuro-Agent** identifies a Large Vessel Occlusion (LVO) in the left Middle Cerebral Artery.

- **Agentic Action:** The agent does not wait for a radiologist to find the scan. It automatically triggers a "Code Stroke" at the regional hub 50 miles away and initiates a secure "Tele-link." While Elena is in the ambulance, the agent is already "Memory-loading" her prior medical history, noting she is on blood thinners—a critical detail for the surgeon.

2. Intra-Procedural Navigation (The GPS)

Elena arrives at the IR suite. Dr. Aris, the interventionalist, begins the mechanical thrombectomy.

- **The Real-Time Fusion:** As Dr. Aris inserts the catheter, the IR Agent overlays Elena's 3D arterial map onto the live, 2D fluoroscopy screen. The agent highlights the "clot zone" in a pulsing blue hue.
- **Pathfinding Reasoning:** The agent detects that Elena's carotid artery is unusually "tortuous" (twisted). It suggests a specific 5-degree tilt of the table and a "steerable" micro-wire path that bypasses the difficult turn. Dr. Aris follows the "digital green line" on the screen, reaching the brain in record time.

3. The "Guardian" Moment (The Safety Net)

During the procedure, as Dr. Aris is deploying the stent-riever to pull out the clot, Elena's blood pressure spikes, and her brain moves slightly due to a cough.

- **Tactile Perception:** The agent senses the movement through the high-speed overhead cameras and the "torque sensors" on the catheter.

- **Rapid Action:** Before Dr. Aris can even react, the agent provides an Audio Alert: *"Vessel wall proximity warning—Stop advancement."* It freezes the navigation overlay to recalibrate for the new head position. This prevents a potential vessel perforation—the most dreaded complication in neuro-intervention.

4. Post-Procedural Assessment (The Closing Loop)

The clot is successfully removed.

- **Automated TICI Scoring:** Within seconds of the final "run" (X-ray injection), the agent analyzes the blood flow. It calculates a TICI 3 Score (perfect re-perfusion) and identifies that all distal branches are now open.

- **The Zero-Click Report:** As Dr. Aris steps away to talk to Elena's family, the agent has already:
    1. Drafted the operative note.
    2. Logged the total "Fluoro Time" (which was 40% lower than average due to the AI navigation).
    3. Sent a "Success Notification" to the neurology ICU to prepare her bed.

Analysis: Why this was an "Agent" and not a "Tool"

Feature	**Traditional AI Tool (2020)**	**Agentic AI (2026)**
Trigger	Human had to open the scan.	Autonomously triggered the alert.
Navigation	Static images on a side monitor.	Live, 3D fused "GPS" on the main screen.
Safety	Retrospective (found errors later).	Proactive (prevented perforation in real-time).
Workflow	Required manual data entry.	Automated the entire reporting and notification cycle.

DIGI HEALTH INSIGHT: The "Interventional Co-Pilot"

The Challenge: The Race Against the Clock During a complex neuro-interventional thrombectomy (stroke treatment), the surgeon must navigate a micro-catheter through tortuous, highly fragile vascular anatomy. "Time is brain," and every second lost to difficult navigation increases the risk of permanent neurological damage or catastrophic vessel perforation.

The Agentic Solution: The Digi Health Digital Co-Pilot The Digi Health IR Agent functioned as an active member of the surgical team, providing a layer of "augmented intelligence" that heightened the surgeon's precision.

- **3D Roadmap Overlay:** The agent projected a real-time, 3D holographic "Roadmap" onto the 2D fluoroscopy screen, dynamically adjusted for the patient's breathing and movement.

- **Predictive Haptics:** The agent monitored the catheter's tension and tip-position, alerting the surgeon to "Vascular Resistance" before a vessel perforation could occur.

- **Autonomous Documentation:** While the surgeon focused on the clot, the agent recorded the entire procedure, logging device timestamps and contrast volumes directly into the EHR via FHIR.

The Result: Redefining the "Golden Hour" The procedure was completed in 18 minutes—a 50% reduction in typical navigation time for this specific anatomy. By eliminating the "3D-to-2D" mental mapping, the surgeon achieved re-perfusion (TICI 3) on the first pass. Furthermore, the "Zero-Click" documentation meant the operative report was finalized and the post-op recovery team was notified before the surgeon had even stepped away from the table. The patient was discharged 48 hours later with a near-complete reversal of symptoms, demonstrating how agentic navigation directly translates to superior clinical outcomes.

Conclusion: The Mission Commander

The transition of the Interventional Radiology suite into a high-tech "cockpit" marks the definitive end of the era of cognitive overload in the operating room. By serving as a Predictive Navigator and a Digital Co-Pilot, the IR Agent of 2026 has effectively solved the "3D-to-2D" mental mapping challenge that has historically burdened even the most skilled surgeons.

In this environment, "Precision" is no longer just a goal—it is a guaranteed clinical standard. The agent's ability to provide real-time haptic feedback, autonomous vascular pathfinding, and "Zero-Touch" orchestration ensures that complex procedures are safer for the patient and significantly less taxing for the clinician.

As we conclude our journey through individual imaging modalities, the IR suite stands as the ultimate proof that an agent is not a replacement for the surgeon, but the essential scaffolding that allows the human "Mission Commander" to operate at the absolute limit of medical possibility.

We have seen how agents see, remember, and act within their respective silos. Now, we move to the final horizon. In Section III: The Autonomous Imaging Department, we will explore how these independent agents converge into a single, unified "Digital Nervous System"—an intelligence that manages the entire lifecycle of the hospital, from the first appointment to the final recovery.

SECTION II WRAP-UP: THE MULTIMODAL SYMPHONY

We have traveled through the corridors of the modern imaging department, from the high-velocity triage of X-ray to the sub-millimeter precision of the Interventional suite. While each modality possesses its own unique physics and clinical pressures, a singular truth has emerged: The Agentic Shift is not an incremental improvement; it is a fundamental re-architecting of how medical data is perceived, reasoned, and acted upon.

The Combined Impact: A High-Level View

By deploying specialized agents across the seven pillars of imaging, the department moves from a collection of "siloed workstations" to a **Unified Intelligence Ecosystem**.

- **Safety & Ethics (The Biological Cost):** Through the "AI Shield" in CT and "Synthetic Fluoro" in IR, we have achieved a 50–70% reduction in radiation exposure. We have proven that higher diagnostic yield no longer requires a higher biological price.

- **The Velocity of Care:** By automating 40% of reporting tasks in Mammography and providing real-time navigation in Ultrasound, we have collapsed the "time-to-diagnosis" from days to minutes.

- **Predictive Precision:** We have transitioned from the reactive (identifying existing pathology) to the proactive (assigning 5-Year Risk Scores in breast health and Ablation Zone Predictions in oncology)

The Modality Matrix Summary

Modality	The Human Role (2026)	The Agent's Primary Value
X-Ray	Quality Gatekeeper	Autonomous Geometric Auditor
CT	Complex Triage Lead	The "AI Shield" & Dose Optimizer
MRI	Functional Interpreter	Synthetic Signal Architect
Ultrasound	Clinical Correlator	Real-Time Navigation Guide
PET/SPECT	Metabolic Strategist	Molecular Noise Subtractor
Mammography	Risk Consultant	The Sentinel (Predictive Memory)
Interventional	Mission Commander	The Digital Co-Pilot (GPS)

SECTION III

THE ORCHESTRATED DEPARTMENT

CHAPTER 11: THE AI ORCHESTRATOR – MANAGING THE MULTI-AGENT ECOSYSTEM

In 2026, the challenge of AI in healthcare has shifted from "How do we build a model?" to "How do we manage the fifty models we already have?" This chapter explores the rise of the AI Orchestrator, the invisible conductor that ensures your specialized agents work in harmony rather than creating a digital cacophony.

Introduction: The Conductor and the Symphony

Imagine a world-class orchestra where every musician is a virtuoso. The violinist is a master of melody, the cellist provides the soul, and the percussionist drives the rhythm. But without a conductor, there is no music—only a chaotic overlap of individual brilliance.

In the radiology department of 2026, we have achieved "agentic virtuosity." We have a Stroke Agent that can spot an occlusion in seconds, a Billing Agent that optimizes revenue, and a Dose Agent that shields the patient from radiation. However, if these agents run in isolation, the result is "Agent Sprawl": conflicting alerts, duplicated data processing, and a radiologist overwhelmed by ten different AI dashboards. The AI Orchestrator is the central intelligence that acts as the conductor, ensuring that the right agent is activated at the right time, with the right context.

Anatomy of the Orchestrator: The Triple-A Framework

The Orchestrator is not just a router; it is a sophisticated meta-agent designed with three core functional layers:

I. The Planner (Intent Analysis)

When a new imaging study arrives, the Orchestrator does not just "push buttons." It analyzes the **clinical intent**. If the order is "Chest CT - Rule out PE," the Planner breaks this down into sub-tasks:

- **Task 1:** Route to the "Vessel Segmentation Agent."
- **Task 2:** Trigger the "Pulmonary Embolism Detection Agent."
- **Task 3:** Cross-reference the "EHR Agent" for recent D-dimer lab results.

- **Task 4:** Alert the "Resident Worklist" if findings are positive.

II. The Dispatcher (Resource Management)

The Dispatcher manages the "Traffic." It understands which agents are high-priority and which are background tasks. It ensures the Stroke Agent gets the highest GPU priority while the Osteoporosis Screening Agent (an opportunistic task) runs during quiet periods. This prevents system latency during critical life-saving procedures.

III. The Verifier (Truth Maintenance)

Perhaps the most critical role in 2026 **is Conflict Resolution. If the "Lung** Nodule Agent" identifies a 5mm spot as "suspicious" but the "Temporal Memory Agent" identifies it as a "stable scar from 2022," the Orchestrator notes the discrepancy. It does not hide the conflict; it flags it for the radiologist with a "Divergent Finding" alert, providing the evidence from both specialized agents side-by-side.

The "Virtual Tumor Board": Orchestration in Action

The power of orchestration is best seen in multidisciplinary care. In 2026, we use Cross-Functional Ecosystems.

Take a complex lung cancer case:

1. The **Radiology Agent** detects a mass and measures its volume.
2. The **Pathology Agent** analyzes the digital biopsy slide and identifies a specific mutation.
3. The **Genomic Agent** sequences the tumor's DNA.
4. The **Orchestrator** pulls these three disparate "opinions" together, queries the latest 2026 clinical guidelines, and drafts a unified "Integrated Diagnostic Report" for the surgeon.

This process, which once took two weeks and three meetings, now happens in the background within hours of the biopsy.

Interoperability: The Model Context Protocol (MCP)

By 2026, the "vendor lock-in" of the early 2020s has been dismantled. The industry has adopted the Model Context Protocol (MCP) and HL7 FHIR as the "universal languages" of healthcare.

- **The Universal Handshake (MCP):** MCP allows an agent built by Company A to share its "reasoning chain" with an Orchestrator built by Company B. When a Radiology Agent identifies a mass, it sends an MCP-wrapped packet containing its confidence score, the specific pixels analyzed, and the clinical guidelines referenced.

- **The Graph-Based Patient (FHIR):** The EHR is no longer a collection of static PDFs; it is a live FHIR-based data graph. Agents "subscribe" to specific FHIR resources. If a lab result for "Creatinine" is updated in the EHR, the CT Agent—via the Orchestrator—immediately receives a notification and adjusts the contrast-injection protocol for the upcoming scan in real-time.

Governance: Who Watches the Watchmen?

With agents managing other agents, human oversight has moved to the Meta-Level.

- **The AI Dashboard:** Department heads no longer just monitor "Turnaround Time" for humans; they monitor Agent Reliability. If the "Stroke Agent" starts showing a 5% drop in accuracy, the Orchestrator flags itself for a "Calibration Review."

- **Human-in-the-Loop Checkpoints:** The Orchestrator is programmed with "Hard Stops." No agent can autonomously order a biopsy or change a medication without a human "Sign-off" in the Orchestrator's interface.

The AI Orchestrator is the "Operating System" of the 2026 hospital. It transforms a collection of high-tech tools into a unified, intelligent partner. By managing the complexity of the multi-agent ecosystem, it allows the human physician to stop being a "Data Coordinator" and return to being a "Healer."

To truly understand how a 2026 hospital functions, we have to look "under the hood" at the invisible plumbing that prevents the AI Orchestrator from becoming a digital black box.

The Technical Bedrock: MCP, FHIR, and the Death of Data Silos

In the early 2020s, AI integration was a nightmare of custom APIs and proprietary "walled gardens." By 2026, two standards have emerged as the "universal translators" for the medical agentic ecosystem.

I. The Model Context Protocol (MCP)

MCP is the breakthrough that allowed for Agentic Fluidity. Previously, if you wanted a "Lung Agent" to talk to a "Billing Agent," you had to write custom code.

- **The Universal Handshake:** MCP provides a standardized way for agents to share their Reasoning Chains. When the Radiology Agent identifies a mass, it does not just send a "Yes" signal; it sends an MCP-wrapped packet containing its confidence score, the specific pixels it analyzed, and the clinical guidelines it referenced.

- **Contextual Persistence:** MCP allows the Orchestrator to maintain a "Shared Memory." If the patient moves from the ER to the ICU, the Orchestrator uses MCP to "hand off" the agent's current state, so the next team does not have to start from scratch.

II. HL7 FHIR (Fast Healthcare Interoperability Resources)

While MCP handles how agents "think" together, FHIR handles how they "access" the patient's life story.

- **The Graph-Based Patient:** In 2026, the Electronic Health Record (EHR) is no longer a collection of PDFs. It is a FHIR-based data graph.
- **Real-Time Subscription:** Agents "subscribe" to specific FHIR resources. If a lab result for "Creatinine" is updated in the EHR, the CT Agent—via the Orchestrator—immediately receives a FHIR notification and adjusts the contrast-injection protocol for the upcoming scan.

Troubleshooting the Orchestrator: When the Conductor Fails

Even the best-designed systems encounter "Edge Cases." In 2026, the most dangerous failure is not a system crash—it is "Orchestration Drift."

I. Conflicting Directives (The "Loop" Problem)

- **The Scenario:** The "Safety Agent" recommends *slowing down* a scan to reduce noise, while the "Efficiency Agent" recommends *speeding up* to clear a backlogged ER.

- **The Solution:** The Orchestrator utilizes a Priority Hierarchy. In 2026, "Clinical Safety" is hard-coded as the apex priority. If two agents conflict, the Orchestrator defaults to the more conservative, safety-oriented path and generates an "Audit Alert" for human review.

II. Hallucination Cascades

- **The Risk:** If a specialized agent "hallucinates" a finding and the Orchestrator accepts it as truth, that error can cascade into the billing, pharmacy, and surgical agents.

- **The "Zero-Trust" Protocol:** To prevent this, 2026 Orchestrators use Ensemble Verification. For any high-stakes finding, the Orchestrator runs the data through a second, differently-architected "Verifier Agent." If the two do not agree, the Orchestrator triggers a "Hard Stop," requiring a human radiologist to "Authenticate" the data before it propagates further.

III. Latency and "Deadlocks"

- **The Technical Failure:** When five agents are trying to access the same high-resolution 3D volume simultaneously, the system can "Deadlock."
- **The Solution:** Modern Orchestrators use Asynchronous Processing. The most time-critical agent (e.g., the Stroke Agent) is given "Atomic Access" to the data, while the secondary agents (e.g., the Research Agent) work on cached, lower-priority versions of the data.

Failure Mode	The Risk	The 2026 Solution
Conflicting Directives	**Safety vs. Efficiency agents suggest opposite scan speeds.**	**Priority Hierarchy: Clinical Safety is hard-coded as the apex priority; defaults to conservative path.**
Hallucination Cascades	**An error in one agent propagates to billing or surgery.**	**Zero-Trust Protocol: High-stakes findings require Ensemble Verification from a second, independent agent.**
Data Deadlocks	**Five agents attempt to access the same 3D volume at once.**	**Asynchronous Processing: Time-critical agents (e.g., Stroke) get "Atomic Access" while others use cached data.**

Conclusion: The "Fail-Safe" Mentality

Troubleshooting the AI Orchestrator in 2026 is less about fixing "bugs" and more about managing Probabilities. We have moved past the era of expecting binary perfection from AI; instead, we have built a system that acknowledges its own limitations. The Orchestrator's true value is not that it never fails, but that it is designed to fail gracefully.

The Orchestrator acts as the ultimate "Fail-Safe," alerting the human physician the moment the digital symphony hits a sour note. It ensures that when an agent drifts or a data conflict arises, the system defaults to safety, transparency, and human oversight.

We have built the engine and connected the wires. We have created a digital nervous system that can see, reason, and coordinate. Now, we must look at the Physical Change. In the next chapter, we explore how these invisible agents are literally reshaping the bricks and mortar of the hospital—moving from "Imaging Departments" to "Diagnostic Command Centers."

CHAPTER 12: THE COMMAND CENTER – THE NEW RADIOLOGY READING ROOM

In 2026, the transition of the radiology workspace is complete. We have moved from the "Dark Room" era—characterized by isolation and eye strain—to the Command Center era, defined by high-bandwidth collaboration and augmented intelligence. This chapter explores the physical and cognitive architecture of the modern reading room.

The Death of the "Dark Room"

For a century, radiologists worked in near-total darkness to maximize perceived contrast. In 2026, this is a relic. Modern 8K monitors utilize such high luminance and dynamic range that they thrive in ambient daylight.

- **Biophilic Cockpits:** The 2026 Command Center is designed around circadian LED systems and natural light. Research from 2024 proved that this "biophilic" approach reduces late-shift diagnostic errors by 15%.

- **Foveated Rendering:** Using eye-tracking sensors, the workstation renders only the specific area you are looking at in "extreme resolution," reducing GPU heat and cognitive fatigue.

The Agentic Workstation: An Augmented Cockpit

The center of the room is the Unified HUD (Heads-Up Display). Unlike the multi-monitor setups of the 2010s, which forced radiologists to physically turn their necks hundreds of times a day, the 2026 workstation often utilizes a single, ultra-wide curved 8K display.

- **Foveated Rendering:** The workstation uses eye-tracking cameras to determine exactly where the radiologist is looking. It renders that specific area of the image in "extreme resolution" while keeping the periphery in "standard resolution." This saves massive amounts of bandwidth and reduces the cognitive load of the radiologist.
- **The "Sidebar" Agent:** On the edge of the screen, the Orchestrator maintains a live "Pulse List." Instead of a static list of names, this is a dynamic feed. If a patient's status changes in the ICU, their scan moves up the list in real-time, pulsing with a subtle orange glow.

- **Haptic Feedback:** Some advanced stations utilize "Haptic Mice" or "Ultrasonic Mid-Air Haptics." When the radiologist's cursor passes over a calcified edge or a dense mass, they feel a subtle "resistance" or "click," adding a tactile dimension to the visual search.

Ambient Intelligence and Notification Logic

The greatest enemy of the 2020s radiologist was "Alert Fatigue." In 2026, we have solved this through Ambient Notification.

- **Spatial Audio:** Instead of a generic "beep," the Command Center uses directional sound. An urgent alert from the ER might sound like it is coming from the left, while a routine billing query sounds like it is coming from the far right. The radiologist "perceives" the urgency without having to stop their current task.

- **Gaze-Aware Interruptions:** The Orchestrator "waits" for a break in the radiologist's gaze before presenting a non-urgent notification. If the doctor is deeply focused on a complex spine CT, the agent suppresses all but life-critical interruptions until the doctor leans back or looks away from the screen.

The Collaborative Core: Virtual and Physical

The Command Center acts as the "Air Traffic Control" for the entire hospital.

- **The "Glass Wall" Consultation:** Using high-definition transparent displays, radiologists can initiate a "Face-to-Face" with a surgeon in the OR. Both can see the same 3D model of the patient, and both can "draw" on the image in real-time.

- **AI-Language Translation:** If a radiologist in London is consulting on a case in Tokyo, the Communication Agent performs real-time, low-latency voice translation, ensuring that nuances of "suspected malignancy" are not lost in translation.

Ergonomics and the "Pilot" Protocol

To manage the psychological shift toward "Supervisory Interpretation," Command Centers have adopted aviation-style Checklist Protocols.

- **Active Verification:** Every 20 minutes, the workstation might prompt a "Calibration Check." The radiologist must confirm a small finding to ensure they have not fallen into "Automation Bias"—blindly trusting the AI's suggestions.

- **Physical Movement:** The "Smart Chair" tracks the radiologist's posture. If the agent detects signs of physical fatigue (slumping or decreased blink rate), it suggests a "micro-break" or automatically transitions the desk to standing mode to re-energize the clinician.

Summary: A Workspace for the Future

The 2026 Command Center is more than a room with computers. It is a Human-Machine **Interface** designed to amplify human expertise. By removing the physical and cognitive friction of the old "Dark Room" era, we have created a space where the radiologist can finally work at the speed of thought.

In 2026, the Command Center is no longer tethered to the hospital's basement. The same "Orchestrator" that manages the hospital's massive GPU clusters now extends its reach to the suburban home and the rural satellite office, ensuring that the "Pilot" can fly the mission from anywhere.

The Distributed Cockpit: Teleradiology in 2026

The "Home-Based Command Center" is the final frontier of the digitized department. By 2026, the technical gap between the hospital and the home has vanished, thanks to two critical advancements:

- **The Virtualized GPU (vGPU):** High-end 3D rendering and AI inference no longer happen on the local PC. The home workstation acts as a "Thin Client," while the heavy lifting is done by the hospital's central "Agentic Cloud." This allows a radiologist to manipulate a 4,000-slice CT scan with zero latency over a standard fiber-optic home connection.

- **Biometric Security & Privacy:** In 2026, a home-based Command Center is secured by Continuous Biometric Authentication. The system uses infrared facial recognition and gaze-tracking to ensure that only the credentialed radiologist is viewing the screen. If an unauthorized person enters the room, the AI Agent instantly "blurs" the patient data on the monitor.

Case Study: A "Day in the Life" (Sarah Chen, MD)

08:00 AM – The "Warm-Start" Login

Dr. Sarah Chen logs into her home workstation. The Orchestrator greets her with a "Morning Brief." Instead of a raw list of 100 cases, the agent shows a "Decision Map."

> *"Good morning, Sarah. I have pre-processed 42 cases. 38 are routine and have drafted reports waiting for your sign-off. I have flagged 4 cases for immediate review: two suspected strokes and one complex oncology staging with conflicting AI opinions."*

09:30 AM – The "Reasoning Duel"

Sarah opens a chest CT. The Nodule Agent has flagged a lung spot as "High Risk," but the Longitudinal Memory Agent has cross-referenced a 2023 X-ray from a different hospital and identified it as a stable granuloma. Sarah enters the "Reasoning Duel" mode. She views the 2023 and 2026 images side-by-side, overlaid with the agent's heatmaps. She agrees with the Memory Agent, "Overrules" the Nodule Agent, and the Report Agent instantly updates the draft to reflect a "Benign Finding."

11:00 AM – The Virtual "Ping"

While Sarah is reading a routine MRI, her "Ambient HUD" pulses a soft blue on the right side. It is Dr. Aris from the IR Suite (Chapter 10). He is in the middle of a difficult catheterization and needs a second look at the 3D vascular anatomy. Sarah taps her "Collaborate" button. A window opens on her HUD showing the live surgical feed. Using gesture control, she "rotates" the 3D model on Dr. Aris's screen, pointing out a hidden vessel branch. "There it is, Aris. Take the left turn."

01:00 PM – The Patient Consultation

The Communication Agent notifies Sarah that a patient, Mr. Miller, has a high level of anxiety regarding his recent scan results. Sarah enters a "Consultation Pod" (virtually). She shares a "Simplified View" with Mr. Miller via a secure link. The AI has converted the dense medical jargon into a 3D visual of his heart. Sarah explains the finding, the AI provides real-time captions and translations, and Mr. Miller leaves the call feeling empowered rather than confused.

04:00 PM – The Seamless Handoff

As Sarah prepares to log off, the Orchestrator prepares the "Night-Shift Handoff." It summarizes the "Pending" cases and the reasoning steps she took on the complex oncology case. She signs off, and her entire digital workspace is mirrored to the "Night Command Center" in London, where her colleague is just beginning their day.

Time	Event	Agentic Action
08:00	The Warm-Start	The Orchestrator presents a "Decision Map" instead of a worklist, highlighting 4 "Reasoning Duels" needing human intervention.
09:30	The Reasoning Duel	Sarah overrules a Nodule Agent after the Memory Agent pulls a 2023 X-ray proving the spot is a stable scar.
11:00	Virtual "Ping"	Sarah "teleports" into the IR suite via a HUD overlay to guide a surgeon through a hidden vessel branch in real-time.
13:00	Patient Consultation	Sarah shares a "Simplified View" with a patient; the AI converts jargon into 3D visuals to explain a heart finding.
16:00	Global Handoff	The workspace mirrors to the Night Command Center in London, including all "Reasoning Chains" for pending cases.

Conclusion: The Empowerment of the Professional

The 2026 Command Center has not replaced the radiologist; it has replaced the drudgery. By automating the search, the reporting, and the logistics, the Command Center allows the physician to spend their time where it matters most: on the difficult "edge cases," the surgical collaborations, and the human connection with their patients.

In the agentic era, we have finally reconciled the machine's speed with the human's wisdom. As we look to the final horizon of this book, we see that the Command Center is not just a room—it is the heartbeat of a new, Value-Based healthcare economy. We have optimized the *where* and the *how*; now, we must examine the *why* as we look toward a future of proactive, personalized wellness for all.

CHAPTER 13: THE ETHICAL COMPASS – BIAS, LIABILITY, AND THE BLACK BOX

In 2026, the ethical landscape of medical imaging has shifted from philosophical debate to "hard-coded" regulation. As AI agents move from being tools to becoming autonomous decision-partners, the industry has had to reconcile the speed of innovation with the immutable requirements of medical ethics: justice, non-maleficence, and accountability.

The Death of the "Black Box": Explainable AI (XAI)

The greatest ethical crisis of early medical AI was the "Black Box" problem—the inability of a machine to explain *why* it reached a specific conclusion. In 2026, the Right to Explanation is a legally mandate.

Modern agents utilize Transparent Reasoning Chains. When an agent identifies a suspicious lesion, the radiologist can click on a "Reasoning Tree." The agent then provides a breakdown of its logic:

- **Visual Evidence:** Highlighting the specific texture and boundary irregularities.
- **Comparative Evidence:** Displaying three similar "verified" cases from its memory.
- **Clinical Evidence:** Citing the specific 2025 guidelines (e.g., PI-RADS v3) that influenced the score.
-

This "Show Your Work" protocol prevents the radiologist from becoming a "rubber stamp" and ensures that if a machine makes a mistake, the human can identify the specific logical flaw (e.g., "The agent is mistaking surgical hardware for a calcification").

Algorithmic Bias and the "Equity Guardrail"

In the early 2020s, it was discovered that many AI models were trained on "convenience data"—largely from affluent, urban, Western populations. This led to Diagnostic Drift, where accuracy plummeted for patients from marginalized or rural backgrounds.

By 2026, the AI Orchestrator acts as an Equity Auditor. It performs "Continuous Bias Monitoring" across four key pillars:

1. **Demographic Parity:** Does the agent perform equally well across different ethnicities and ages?
2. **Anatomical Variation:** Can the agent handle diverse body types and BMI levels?
3. **Site-Specific Bias:** Has the agent "over-fitted" to the specific quirks of one hospital's scanning hardware?
4. **Socioeconomic Context:** Does the agent's recommendation take into account the patient's access to follow-up care?

If an agent's performance drops for a specific subgroup, the Orchestrator automatically "de-rates" the agent's confidence score for those cases and triggers a manual human-led audit.

The Liability Loop: The "Last Clear Chance" Doctrine

The legal world in 2026 has introduced the **"Shared Responsibility Framework."** For years, the question was: "If the AI misses a tumor, who gets sued?"

The 2026 framework operates on three levels:

- **The Radiologist's Burden:** If the AI flags a finding and the radiologist dismisses it without a documented reason, the radiologist holds 100% liability.
- **The Vendor's Burden:** If the AI has a "Systemic Failure" (e.g., a software bug that renders certain pixels invisible), the manufacturer is held strictly liable.
- **The "Joint Venture":** If the error is an "Interpretive Edge Case"—a subtle finding that both a reasonable human and a high-performing AI might miss—the liability is shared between the hospital and the insurance carrier, recognizing that medicine is an inherently probabilistic science.

Automation Bias and the "Human-in-the-Loop"

Perhaps the most subtle ethical threat is **Automation Bias**—the human tendency to trust the machine more than one's own eyes. To combat this, 2026 Command Centers have implemented **"Blind Verification"** tests.

Once a week, the Orchestrator presents the radiologist with a "Challenge Case"—a scan where the agent has intentionally hidden its findings. This forces the radiologist to perform a completely manual search, ensuring their diagnostic muscles do not "atrophy" from over-reliance on the agent.

Data Sovereignty and the "Right to Forget"

In an era where agents "learn" from every scan they see, the patient's privacy is under constant threat of being "digitally absorbed."

- **Differential Privacy:** 2026 agents use mathematical "noise" to ensure that while the agent can learn the *pattern* of a disease, it can never "re-identify" the specific patient's identity.

- **The Digital Will:** Patients now have a "Digital Sovereignty" setting in their EHR. They can choose to allow their data to be used for "Clinical Care" but opt out of "Agentic Training," effectively preventing their biological data from becoming part of a corporation's global model.

The 2026 radiologist is no longer just a "looker at pictures." They have become the Ethical Steward of the digital department. Their role is to ensure that the speed and power of the agentic ecosystem never come at the cost of the patient's dignity, privacy, or right to a fair diagnosis.

Adversarial Attacks: Tricking the Digital Eye

In 2026, the greatest threat to medical AI is not a software bug, but a deliberate "illusion." **Adversarial Attacks** use targeted manipulations of image data that are invisible to the human eye but catastrophic for the machine.

- **Pixel-Level Sabotage (The Invisible Tumor):** A hacker can introduce microscopic "noise" into a CT scan. This noise is mathematically calculated to exploit the agent's neural network. By changing just a few dozen pixels (imperceptible to the human eye), an attacker can trick the "Cancer Agent" into seeing a non-existent malignant tumor or, more dangerously, "hiding" a real one. Research shows that a perturbation of just 0.004 (on a 0-1 scale) can drop a model's accuracy from 95% to below 25%, causing it to "hide" a real lung nodule or see a non-existent tumor

- **The "GAN-based" Erasure:** Using Generative Adversarial Networks (the same tech that powers Deepfakes), attackers can "reconstruct" a patient's scan to remove evidence of a heart condition or an aneurysm. In 2026, this is identified as a major risk for Insurance Fraud (to lower premiums) or Political Sabotage (to alter the medical records of a public figure).

Digital Watermarking and Proactive Defense

To combat these threats, 2026 hospitals have moved beyond standard firewalls to Agentic Cybersecurity.

- **Cryptographic Watermarking:** Every scan is "stamped" with a digital signature at the moment of capture. If a single pixel is altered between the scanner and the reading room, the Orchestrator identifies a "Hash Mismatch" and flags the image as compromised.

- **Adversarial Training:** AI agents are now trained on "Antidote" datasets. During their development, they are intentionally fed millions of hacked images. This teaches the agent to recognize the mathematical "signatures" of an attack, making the model "Certified Robust."

Conclusion: The Ethical Steward

The 2026 radiologist has transcended the role of a "looker at pictures." In the agentic era, they have become the Ethical Steward—the high-level governor of a digital department. Their primary mission is to ensure that the unprecedented speed and predictive power of the ecosystem never come at the cost of the patient's dignity, privacy, or right to an equitable diagnosis.

As the "Human-in-the-Loop," the radiologist acts as the final arbiter of truth, resolving the "Reasoning Duels" between agents and defending the clinical workflow against Adversarial Drift. By mastering the "Triple-A" framework of orchestration and the "Zero-Trust" protocols of cybersecurity, the 2026 clinician ensures that AI remains a partner in healing rather than a black box of liability.

We have now secured the technology, the architecture, and the ethics. But for whom have we built this symphony? In the final section, The Patient's Journey, we step out of the Command Center and into the lives of the people we serve. We will see how this "invisible" technology manifests as a visible miracle: a world where no patient is ever "lost" in the system again.

SECTION IV

THE BLUEPRINT FOR IMPLEMENTATION

CHAPTER 14: THE LIFECYCLE OF THE AI AGENT

In **Section IV**, we move away from "what" the technology does and focus on the high-stakes "how" of making it work. Implementing agentic AI is not a standard software install; it is a clinical integration project that requires a lifecycle approach.

Implementing an AI agent in a radiology department in 2026 follows a rigorous seven-phase lifecycle. This ensures that the agent is not just a "bolt-on" tool but a seamless part of the clinical nervous system.

Planning: The Pain-Point Charter

Before a single line of code is written or a vendor is contacted, the department must define the Clinical Objective.

- **Defining the Use Case:** Is the agent solving a throughput issue (e.g., bone age turnaround) or a safety issue (e.g., pulmonary embolism triage)?

- **Stakeholder Alignment:** Establishing a "Triple-A" committee (Administrative, AI-Technical, and Anatomical/Clinical) to ensure the agent meets the needs of IT, the budget, and the doctors.

- **KPI Baseline:** Measuring current performance metrics (e.g., "Mean Time to Notify for Critical Findings") to establish the "Before AI" benchmark.

Development: Training with Context

Generic models are a relic of 2023. Modern development focuses on Retrieval-Augmented Generation (RAG) and Model Tuning using local hospital parameters.

- **Data Curation:** Selecting "Gold Standard" datasets that include the specific scanners and patient demographics of the local hospital to prevent "Model Drift."
- **Integration Planning:** Designing the agent to communicate via FHIR and DICOMweb standards so it can "read" the EHR and "write" to the PACS (Picture Archiving and Communication System) without custom middleware.

Testing: The "Shadow Mode" Protocol

In 2026, we never "flip a switch" on a new agent. We use Shadow Mode.

- **Parallel Processing:** The agent runs in the background on every live case. It generates its findings, but they are hidden from the clinical staff.

- **Retrospective Comparison:** After 30 days, a "Turing Review" is conducted. The agent's findings are compared to the final human-signed reports. If the agreement rate is >98% and no critical "misses" occurred, the agent moves to the next phase.

Production Rollout: The Orchestrated Launch

The transition from "Shadow" to "Live" is done in waves.

- **The "Champion" Phase:** A small group of "Super-User" radiologists uses the agent for one week, providing real-time feedback on UI/UX friction.

- **Silent Action:** The agent begins performing non-diagnostic tasks first (e.g., auto-populating patient history or pre-fetching prior scans) before it is allowed to offer diagnostic suggestions.

Evaluation: Measuring the "AI Dividend"

Once live, the agent is continuously evaluated against the KPIs set in Phase 1.

- **Clinical Impact:** Did the "Time to Treatment" for stroke patients actually decrease?

- **Financial Impact:** Did the agent reduce the "Rejection Rate" for insurance claims by improving documentation accuracy?
- **Physician Wellness:** A "Burnout Survey" is administered to see if the agent reduced the "Clicks-per-Case" for the radiologists.

Administration: The "Agentic Governance"

Managing an agent requires a new type of hospital administrator: the AI Steward.

- **Registry Management:** Maintaining a "Living Risk Register" of every agent, its current version, its "Last Calibration" date, and its known failure modes.

- **Audit Trails:** Ensuring every agentic decision is logged. If a patient asks, *"Why was my scan prioritized this way?"* the administrator must be able to pull the agent's MCP (Model Context Protocol) reasoning chain.

Upgrade and Retirement: Managing "Model Decay"

AI agents are not static; they "decay" as hospital equipment is upgraded or clinical guidelines change.

- **The Continuous Improvement Loop:** When a new version of the agent is released (e.g., "Mammography Agent v2.1"), it enters a mini-shadow mode (Phase 3) before replacing v2.0.

- **Decommissioning:** If an agent's accuracy falls below the human baseline or if a more capable multi-modal agent renders it redundant, it is "gracefully retired," ensuring all its historical "Memory" is securely archived.

Conclusion: The Disciplined Path to Value

The lifecycle of an AI agent is a move from experimental curiosity to operational infrastructure. By 2026, we have learned that the success of AI is not determined by the complexity of the neural network, but by the discipline of the integration.

Managing this lifecycle ensures that the "Digital Co-Pilot" remains a reliable partner, rather than a liability. When an agent is planned with intent, tested in the shadows, and retired with grace, it stops being a "tool" and becomes an enduring part of the hospital's legacy.

CHAPTER 15: THE INTEGRATION STACK – FHIR, DICOMWEB, AND API SECURITY

In Chapter 15, we move from the high-level roadmap to the "plumbing" that makes an agentic radiology department possible. By 2026, the industry has abandoned messy, custom-coded integrations in favor of a standardized Integration Stack. This stack ensures that AI agents can "talk" to scanners, records, and each other with zero friction and maximum security.

The Core Infrastructure: The "Big Three" Standards

To operate autonomously, an AI agent requires three standardized interfaces to interact with the hospital's digital environment.

- **DICOMweb (The Image Gateway):** Traditional DICOM was designed for high-bandwidth local networks. DICOMweb is the modern, RESTful evolution. It allows agents to "query" and "retrieve" specific image slices via standard web protocols (WADO-RS, QIDO-RS). This is essential for agents running in the cloud or as microservices.
-
- **HL7 FHIR (The Clinical Context):** As discussed in Section III, FHIR is the language of the EHR. An agent uses FHIR to pull "Social Determinants of Health," recent lab results, or allergy profiles to provide a "Context-Aware" diagnosis.
-
- **Model Context Protocol (MCP):** The newest addition to the stack in 2026. MCP acts as the "Universal Translator" between different AI models. It allows a "Stroke Agent" to hand off its findings to a "Billing Agent" without losing the underlying reasoning or metadata.

The Orchestration Layer: API Gateways

In a 2026 department, you do not connect an agent directly to the PACS. Instead, you use an AI API Gateway.

- **Traffic Management:** The gateway ensures that an intensive 3D-processing agent does not "choke" the network during peak ER hours.

- **Standardization:** It converts legacy HL7 v2 messages from older hospital systems into the modern FHIR resources that agents can understand.

- **Versioning:** It manages different versions of agents simultaneously, allowing for the "Shadow Mode" testing described in Chapter 14.

Enterprise-Grade Security: Zero-Trust for AI

Because agents are autonomous, they represent a new "Attack Surface." By 2026, security is handled through a Zero-Trust Architecture.

- **Machine Identity Management (IAM):** Every AI agent is treated as a "Digital Employee." It has its own unique credentials, specific permissions (e.g., "Read-only access to Chest X-rays"), and an expiration date for its access tokens.

- **End-to-End Encryption:** Data is encrypted at rest (in the database) and in transit. Using mTLS (Mutual TLS), the agent and the server must both prove their identity before a single pixel is exchanged.

- **Audit Logging:** Every time an agent accesses a file, a permanent, tamper-proof log is created. In the event of a breach or a clinical error, the administration can see exactly which agent accessed which file at what microsecond.

Implementation Detail: The "Sidecar" Deployment

One of the most efficient implementation patterns in 2026 is the Sidecar Deployment.

Instead of rewriting the PACS software to include AI, the AI agent runs as a "Sidecar" container. It "sniffs" the incoming DICOM traffic, performs its analysis in parallel, and then "injects" its findings back into the radiologist's viewer as a standardized DICOM Structured Report (SR) or an Overlaid GSPS (Grayscale Softcopy Presentation State).

Technical Deep-Dive: The "FHIR Observation" Loop

We moved beyond the conceptual to the "wires and pipes" of the department. Now, we perform a technical deep-dive into the most critical transaction in the 2026 radiology workflow: How an AI agent converts an image finding into a medical record.

This process is known as Bridging the Semantic Gap—moving from a 3D pixel coordinate in a DICOM image to a structured "Observation" in a FHIR database.

By 2026, we have moved past simple PDF reports. Today, AI agents are "Primary Authors" of structured clinical data. When an agent finds a lung nodule, it does not just draw a box; it triggers a sophisticated data mapping sequence.

A. The Translation: From DICOM SR to FHIR

Historically, radiology findings were locked in DICOM Structured Reports (SR)—a format radiologists use but the rest of the hospital cannot read. The 2026 AI Agent acts as a real-time translator.

- **The Trigger:** The agent completes its pixel analysis and generates a DICOM SR.

- **The Mapping:** An Integration Agent instantly maps the DICOM tags to the FHIR Observation Resource. For example, the DICOM tag for "Long Axis Measurement" is mapped to Observation.valueQuantity.

B. Anatomy of an Agent-Generated FHIR Observation

In 2026, an AI-authored observation is much richer than a human note. It includes critical "Metadata" that ensures transparency.

FHIR Element	Data Injected by AI Agent
status	preliminary (Until human sign-off)
category	imaging
code	LOINC Code (e.g., 24611-6 for Chest CT)
valueQuantity	The actual measurement (e.g., 8.2 mm)
interpretation	High Risk (Based on AI risk model)

FHIR Element	Data Injected by AI Agent
device	Reference to the specific AI Model & Version (e.g., Nodule-Agent-v4.2)
derivedFrom	Reference to the specific ImagingStudy and ImageInstance

C. Provenance: The "AI-Assisted" Label

One of the major implementation requirements of 2026 is Provenance. In the FHIR resource, we use the meta.security or Provenance resource to flag that this data was authored by an AI.

- **The Verifier:** The FHIR resource includes a reference to the Verifier (the Human Radiologist). The observation is not considered "Final" until the radiologist's digital signature is attached to the FHIR resource, creating a permanent record of the Human-AI collaboration.

D. Closing the Loop: The "Observation-to-Order" Action

The true power of 2026 agentic implementation is Automatic Actionability.

Once the FHIR Observation is written to the EHR:

1. **The Clinical Decision Support (CDS) Hook:** The EHR "sees" the new observation.

2. **The Logic Gate:** If the Observation says *"Lung Nodule > 6mm"* and the patient is a smoker, the system automatically drafts a ServiceRequest (Order) for a follow-up CT in 6 months.

3. **Human Verification:** The radiologist sees a pop-up: *"Agent suggests 6-month follow-up based on BTS Guidelines. Approve?"* One click, and the entire care pathway is secured.

Conclusion: The Invisible Foundation

The Integration Stack is the silent engine of the 2026 hospital. By standardizing how agents see (DICOMweb), think (MCP), and record (FHIR), we have eliminated the data silos that once choked medical progress. This technical bedrock ensures that a finding in the radiology suite doesn't just sit in a folder—it triggers an immediate, secure, and verifiable care pathway.

CHAPTER 16: THE FINANCIAL MODEL – ROI, REIMBURSEMENT, AND THE AI DIVIDEND

In this chapter, we address the "bottom line." In 2026, the question is no longer whether AI agents work, but how they are funded and how they generate value. The financial implementation of agentic AI marks a shift from viewing software as a "cost center" to viewing it as a "revenue and efficiency engine."

The Shift in Procurement: From CapEx to OpEx

Historically, hospitals bought software as a massive upfront Capital Expenditure (CapEx). In 2026, the rapid evolution of models makes this obsolete.

- **The "SaaS + Success" Model:** Most departments now use an Operating Expenditure (OpEx) model. Hospitals pay a base subscription for the Orchestrator and a "Success-Based" fee for specialized agents. If the agent does not meet its KPI (e.g., reducing turnaround time by 20%), the fee is discounted.

- **The "Per-Click" vs. "Value-Based" Tiers:** Low-stakes agents (e.g., auto-measuring a bone) are often billed per-study, while high-impact agents (e.g., early stroke detection) are billed based on the "clinical outcome" or hospital stay reduction.

Capturing the "AI Dividend"

The Return on Investment (ROI) for agentic AI in 2026 is measured in three distinct "dividends":

- **The Efficiency Dividend:** By automating 80% of the "pre-reporting" (measurements, history, and template drafting), a radiologist can handle 25% more cases without increasing their work hours. This reduces the need for expensive locum (temporary) staffing.

- **The Leakage Dividend:** AI agents excel at finding "incidentalomas"—small findings on a scan that need follow-up. By automatically tracking these and scheduling follow-up appointments, the hospital ensures patients stay within their system for future care, capturing revenue that previously "leaked" out when patients forgot to follow up.

- **The Quality Dividend:** Reduction in diagnostic errors leads to lower medical malpractice insurance premiums and avoids the massive costs associated with "never-events" (like a missed critical bleed).

Reimbursement in 2026: The "AI CPT Codes"

By 2026, the regulatory landscape has finally caught up.

- **New Technology Add-on Payments (NTAP):** Medicare and private insurers now provide specific add-on payments for procedures where an "FDA-Cleared Agentic Assistant" was used to improve patient outcomes.

- **Value-Based Contracts:** Large health systems now sign contracts with insurers where they are paid for "Lives Managed" rather than "Procedures Done." In this model, the AI agent is the primary tool for keeping costs low by catching diseases at Stage 1 instead of Stage 4.

Evaluating Total Cost of Ownership (TCO)

Implementation is not just the license fee. A 2026 budget must include:

- **Inference Costs:** The electricity and GPU "compute" required to run the models (either on-premise or in the cloud).

- **Maintenance & Monitoring:** The salary of the AI Steward (from Chapter 14) who manages the agentic ecosystem.

- **Integration Overhead:** The cost of the FHIR/DICOMweb "pipes" described in Chapter 15.

Summary: The Profitability of Precision

In 2026, a radiology department without AI agents is financially unsustainable. The "Precision ROI" of agentic AI allows hospitals to survive in a high-inflation, low-reimbursement environment by doing more with less, while simultaneously improving the quality of the care they provide.

CHAPTER 17: CHANGE MANAGEMENT & STAFF TRAINING – FROM ANXIETY TO ADOPTION

In Chapter 17, we address the final and most vital component of any technological shift: the Human Factor. Even the most advanced AI agent in 2026 is useless if the clinical staff views it with suspicion or if it disrupts the delicate social fabric of the reading room.

The Psychology of the "Agentic Shift"

The introduction of agents is often met with two conflicting emotions: Fear (of replacement) and Fatigue (of yet another software update). In 2026, we manage this through a "Partnership Narrative."

- **Role Redefinition:** We explicitly re-frame the radiologist's role. They are moving from "Primary Searcher" to "Clinical Diagnostic Conductor." The agent is presented as a "Super-Resident" that handles the grunt work, not a competitor for the doctor's seat.

- **Addressing Deskilling:** A major concern in 2026 is "Skill Atrophy." Implementation plans must include "Manual Days" or "Blind Challenges" (as discussed in Section III, Chapter 16) to ensure staff feel their expertise is still being sharpened, not dulled.

The "Champion" Model: Identifying Local Pilots

Implementation never happens top-down; it happens peer-to-peer.

- **Selecting AI Champions:** We identify early adopters within the department—often a mix of tech-savvy residents and respected senior faculty—to serve as "AI Champions."

- **The Feedback Loop:** Champions are the first to use the agent in "Shadow Mode." They provide the "Linguistic Calibration," ensuring the agent's drafted reports sound like a doctor from *their* hospital, not a generic computer.

The 2026 Training Curriculum

Training for agentic AI is no longer a one-day workshop; it is a multi-modal "Upskilling" journey.

- **AI Literacy Modules:** Staff are trained on the "Why" behind the "How." This includes basic training on Probabilistic Reasoning (understanding that an 85% confidence score is not a "Yes/No" but a statistical weight).

- **Adversarial Awareness:** Training staff to recognize "Edge Cases" where agents might hallucinate or struggle (e.g., unusual surgical hardware or motion artifacts).

- **The Simulation Lab:** Using a "Sandbox" environment where radiologists can "break" the agent in a safe space, testing its limits on difficult, anonymized cases before going live with real patients.

Overcoming Resistance: The "Quick Win" Strategy

To win over skeptics, implementation starts with Low-Stakes, High-Relief tasks.

- **Auto-Documentation First:** Before the agent is allowed to suggest a diagnosis, it is used to automate the most hated part of the job: the "pajama time" spent on clinical history and template normalization.

- **The "Safety Net" Reveal:** During the Shadow phase, we show skeptics cases they *missed* that the agent *caught*. Seeing the agent act as a "Guardian" against a potentially fatal error is the single most effective way to turn a skeptic into an advocate.

Evaluating Cultural Health

Implementation is only successful if the "Vibe" of the department remains healthy.

- **The Friction Metric:** We track "Clicks-per-Case" and "Time-on-Screen." If these go up after AI implementation, the agent has failed the change management test.

- **Staff Wellness Surveys:** Regularly measuring "Cognitive Load" to ensure the Orchestrator is successfully filtering noise rather than adding to it.

Summary: The Human-Centric Outcome

By 2026, the success of AI is measured not by its processing speed, but by its impact on Staff Wellness.

Metric	Goal for 2026 Implementation
Cognitive Load	**25% Reduction** in "perceived mental exhaustion" per shift.
Friction Metric	**Zero increase** in "clicks-per-case" after the first 30 days.
Patient Time	**15% Increase** in time available for direct clinician-patient consultation.

Ultimately, change management in the agentic era is about moving from "using a tool" to "leading a team." When the staff feels empowered as the governors of the technology, the department moves from a state of anxiety to a culture of high-performance innovation.

Conclusion: The New Horizon

We have explored the agents, the architecture, the economics, and the people. We have built a blueprint for a department that is faster, safer, and more human.

But 2026 is just the beginning. As we close this book, we look toward **2030**—an era where the "Orchestrator" doesn't just manage a department, but begins to predict and prevent disease before the patient even enters the scanner. The symphony is playing; it is time for the conductor to take the stage.

CHAPTER 18: THE MODALITY-SPECIFIC IMPLEMENTATION LIFECYCLE

In 2026, the implementation of agentic AI is not a "one-size-fits-all" software deployment. Because the physics and clinical workflows of CT, MRI, Ultrasound, and X-ray differ fundamentally, the 7-Phase Lifecycle must be tailored to the specific needs of each modality and the human team operating them.

This chapter details how the 7 phases—Planning, Development, Testing, Rollout, Evaluation, Administration, and Upgrade—are executed across the seven core imaging modalities.

Computed Tomography (CT): The "High-Velocity" Path

Focus: Triage, Throughput, and Dose Optimization.

- **Planning:** The team (Radiologist + CT Tech) identifies bottlenecks in ER turnaround times.
- **Development:** The focus is on Low-Dose Reconstruction. The agent is trained to "clean" images taken with minimal radiation.
- **Testing:** "Shadow Mode" compares AI triage of intracranial hemorrhages against human "Stat" reads to ensure zero false negatives.
- **Rollout:** The CT Technologist is the primary user, utilizing the agent to auto-reconstruct slices before the patient leaves the gantry.
- **Evaluation:** Success is measured by the "Door-to-Intervention" time for stroke patients.
- **Administration:** Monitoring for "Scanner Drift" if a new X-ray tube is installed.
- **Upgrade:** Seamlessly moving to a "Spectral CT" agent as hardware evolves.

Magnetic Resonance Imaging (MRI): The "Quality & Speed" Path

Focus: Scan Time Reduction and Motion Correction.

- **Planning:** Focuses on reducing the "Patient Backlog" by shortening 45-minute scans to 15 minutes.

- **Development:** Utilizing Generative AI to create "Synthetic Sequences" (e.g., creating a T2-weighted image from a T1 input).
- **Testing:** Assessing if AI-accelerated images maintain the same diagnostic "texture" as traditional slow-scan images.
- **Rollout:** The MRI Technologist and Nurse are key; they use a "Motion Agent" that alerts them if a patient moves, allowing for immediate correction.
- **Evaluation:** ROI is measured by "Room Utilization Rate" (how many more patients can we fit in an 8-hour shift?).
- **Administration:** Managing "Protocol Consistency" across different MRI magnet strengths (1.5T vs 3T).
- **Upgrade:** Updating the agent as new "High-Gradient" coils are installed.

Ultrasound (US): The "Operator-Assisted" Path

Focus: Guidance, Measurement, and Ergonomics.

- **Planning:** Aims to reduce Sonographer Burnout and repetitive strain injuries from manual measurements.
- **Development:** Focuses on "Anatomical Labeling"—teaching the agent to identify the heart, kidneys, or fetus in real-time.
- **Testing:** Testing "Real-Time Guidance" heatmaps to ensure the agent correctly identifies if a sonographer has "missed a spot" on an organ.
- **Rollout:** The Sonographer is the "Pilot." The agent auto-measures anatomy while the sonographer focuses on patient comfort.
- **Evaluation:** Success is measured by the reduction in "Scanning Time per Organ."
- **Administration:** Managing the "Operator Variability" to ensure the AI provides a consistent baseline regardless of the sonographer's experience level.
- **Upgrade:** Transitioning from 2D to "Real-time 3D/4D" volumetric agents.

X-Ray & Mammography: The "High-Volume" Path

Focus: Positioning, Screening, and Triage.

- **Planning:** Focuses on reducing the "Retake Rate" (scans that have to be redone due to poor positioning).

- **Development:** Training the agent on "Screening Sensitivity"—ensuring it does not miss the smallest calcification in a breast or the faintest fracture.
- **Testing:** A "Double-Blind" test where AI flags are compared against two expert human readers.
- **Rollout:** The Radiologic Technologist (RT) uses a "Positioning Agent" that gives a green/red light for the perfect shot *before* exposure.
- **Evaluation:** Measured by the "Recall Rate" (how many women have to come back for a second mammogram).
- **Administration:** Tracking "Demographic Equity" to ensure the screening agent works equally well across all breast densities and patient ethnicities.
- **Upgrade:** Integrating "Tomosynthesis" (3D X-ray) capabilities into the existing 2D screening agent.

PET and SPECT: The "Molecular & Dosimetry" Path

Focus: Quantification, Radiotracer Optimization, and Dose Reduction.

- **Planning:** The Nuclear Medicine Physician and Health Physicist identify goals to reduce "Isotope Waste" and patient scan times.
- **Development:** Focuses on Low-Count Reconstruction. Agents are trained to generate diagnostic-quality images using 50% less radiotracer, protecting patients from radiation.
- **Testing:** Validating "SUV (Standardized Uptake Value) Consistency." The agent must provide identical quantification results across different scanner manufacturers.
- **Rollout:** The Nuclear Medicine Technologist uses a "Dose-Prediction Agent." Before injection, the AI suggests the exact minimum dose based on the patient's FHIR-derived metabolic profile.
- **Evaluation:** Success is measured by the "Injected Dose per Scan" and the accuracy of the AI-Automated Dosimetry for therapy planning.
- **Administration:** Managing "Isotope Decay Logic"—the agent must autonomously adjust its reasoning and image reconstruction parameters based on the specific half-life of the tracer used (e.g., F-18 (Fluorine-18) and Ga-68 (Gallium-68)).
- **Upgrade:** Integrating "Theranostic Agents" that can simultaneously plan and monitor targeted radionuclide therapy.

Interventional Radiology (IR): The "Real-Time & Sterile" Path

Focus: Navigation, Procedure Simulation, and Radiation Safety.

- **Planning:** The Interventionalist and Lead Nurse focus on reducing "Fluoroscopy Time" (live X-ray exposure) and improving catheter placement accuracy.
- **Development:** Focusing on "Image Fusion". The agent is trained to overlay a 3D pre-op MRI onto a live 2D X-ray feed in real-time.
- **Testing:** "Latency Stress Tests." In the sterile suite, even a 100ms delay in the AI's catheter-tracking signal is unacceptable.
- **Rollout:** The Scrub Nurse and IR Tech utilize "Voice-Controlled AI." Since the doctor is in a sterile gown, the agent responds to voice commands: *"Agent, show me the arterial phase overlay."*
- **Evaluation:** Success is measured by "Total Fluoroscopy Time" and "Contrast Volume Used."
- **Administration:** Managing the "Hybrid Suite Infrastructure"—ensuring the AI agent is synced across the injector, the C-arm, and the patient monitors.
- **Upgrade:** Transitioning to "Robotic-Assisted Agents" where the AI provides haptic resistance to the doctor's hand during delicate wire maneuvers.

Modality Implementation Matrix: The Human/Agent Balance

Modality	Primary Human Driver	7-Phase Focus	2026 Innovation
CT	Radiologist	Triage Speed	Zero-Latency Stroke Alerts
MRI	Tech/Nurse	Sequence Speed	Deep-Learning Reconstruction
Ultrasound	Sonographer	Ergonomics	Real-time Anatomy Mapping
X-Ray	Technologist	Positioning	Pre-exposure "Perfect Shot" AI
PET / SPECT	Nuclear Med Physician	Quantification	Low-Tracer Dose Synthesis
Interventional	IR Radiologist	Real-Time Navigation	3D-Fusion Sterile HUD

Conclusion: The Integrated Team

The implementation lifecycle ensures that by the time an agent reaches Phase 7 (Upgrade), it is no longer "the software"—it is a modality-specific member of the clinical team.

- **Radiologists:** Lead the Planning and Evaluation (The "Scientific Director").
- **Technologists (RT/NM/US):** Lead the Rollout and Testing (The "Pilot").
- **Nurses/APPs:** Lead the Clinical Integration (The "Safety & Care Coordinator"), using AI to stabilize patients and manage critical incidental findings immediately after the scan.

In 2026, the department is no longer a collection of machines; it is a unified intelligence where human expertise and agentic speed are perfectly calibrated to the physics of the image.

SECTION V

THE FUTURE OF AGENTIC MEDICAL IMAGING

CHAPTER 19: THE EVOLUTION OF THE "TOTAL AGENT" – GENERAL MEDICAL INTELLIGENCE (GMI)

As we transition from 2026 toward the end of the decade, the architecture of artificial intelligence in healthcare is undergoing a fundamental phase shift. We are moving away from the era of "Point Solutions"—discrete, narrow agents designed for single tasks like lung nodule detection or bone age assessment—and entering the era of the Total Agent. This evolution represents the birth of General Medical Intelligence (GMI): a unified, multimodal reasoning system that understands the patient not as a series of pixel coordinates, but as a complex, living biological narrative.

The Death of the "Siloed" Agent

In the early 2020s, a radiology department might have utilized twenty different AI models from ten different vendors. Each was a "specialist" that knew nothing of the other. The "Chest Agent" could not see the patient's history of smoking stored in the EHR, and the "Cardiac Agent" had no idea what the "Lab Agent" found in the patient's recent troponin levels.

By 2030, these silos have collapsed. The Total Agent operates on a cross-modal transformer architecture. It processes "tokens" from diverse sources simultaneously: DICOM image pixels, FHIR-based clinical notes, genomic sequences, and real-time biometric streams from wearables. When this agent looks at a CT scan of the heart, it is not just looking for calcification; it is contextualizing that calcification against the patient's genetic predisposition for cardiovascular disease and their recorded exercise frequency. This is "Hyper-Contextualized Diagnosis."

The Pros: The Triple Aim of Agentic Healthcare

The move toward GMI offers a transformative "Triple Aim" that redefines clinical success.

I. Hyper-Personalized Precision

Traditional radiology relies on population averages: "Is this liver larger than the mean for a 50-year-old male?" The Total Agent shifts the benchmark to the individual. By maintaining a Digital Twin (as discussed in Section IV), the AI can perform longitudinal analysis with sub-millimeter precision. It does not ask if a tumor is "large"; it asks if the tumor is behaving exactly as predicted based on the patient's specific immunotherapy regimen. This allows for "Adaptive Therapy"—changing a treatment plan in days rather than months because the Agentic GMI detected a molecular shift in the imaging signature before it became visible to the naked eye.

II. Global Health Equity and the "Democratized Expert"

Perhaps the most profound "Pro" is the ability to export elite-level expertise to under-resourced regions. General Medical Intelligence can be embedded into low-cost, portable hardware. An autonomous Ultrasound "Pod" in a rural village, powered by a Total Agent, can perform a screening that would normally require a fellowship-trained specialist. The GMI guides the local health worker's hand, interprets the findings in real-time, and triggers an automated referral only when necessary. This effectively breaks the geographic "lottery" of healthcare quality.

III. The Restoration of Human Agency

Paradoxically, the "Total Agent" is the greatest tool for humanizing medicine. By automating the "cognitive drudgery"—the hours spent cross-referencing old reports, measuring lesions, and formatting documentation—the AI gives the physician back their most precious resource: Time. In 2030, the radiologist is no longer tethered to a dark room for ten hours a day. They are in the clinic, in the surgical suite, and at the bedside, using the Agent's insights to lead multidisciplinary care teams.

The Cons: The Systemic Risks of Autonomy

The rise of GMI brings with it "Black Swan" risks that could destabilize the very foundation of medical practice if not managed with extreme rigor.

I. The Skill Atrophy Paradox (The "Pilot" Problem)

As GMI becomes more reliable, the "Human-in-the-Loop" becomes increasingly passive. We face the risk of a generation of "Dashboard Physicians" who can verify an AI's conclusion but cannot perform the fundamental "manual" deduction required if the system fails. If a catastrophic cyber-attack or solar flare were to take the Agentic Mesh offline, would the 2030 workforce have the "muscle memory" to read a complex trauma CT without their digital "autopilot"? This "Cognitive Atrophy" is the hidden cost of convenience.

II. Algorithmic "Gaslighting" and Reasoning Hallucinations

While early AI "hallucinated" in obvious ways (like seeing a tooth in a lung), GMI hallucinations are much more dangerous because they are logical. A Total Agent might provide a perfectly reasoned argument for a diagnosis, citing three different papers and two "similar" cases from its memory, all while being fundamentally wrong due to a "reasoning loop" error. Because the explanation sounds so professional and "human," the clinician may suffer from Automation Bias, ignoring their own gut instinct in favor of the machine's eloquent but flawed deduction.

III. Data Colonization and the "Privacy Debt"

To maintain its "Total" status, GMI requires a constant, unceasing flow of live patient data. This creates an ethical "Privacy Debt." Who owns the "insight" derived from a patient's unique biological signature? If an Agent learns a new way to detect Alzheimer's by studying a specific patient's brain scans, does that patient own a piece of the resulting algorithm? The risk of "Data Colonization" by large tech corporations—where the most intimate details of human biology are harvested to build proprietary GMI—remains a primary concern for 2030 governance.

IV. The Liability "Gray Zone"

As agents move from "suggesting" to "acting" (e.g., the AI Orchestrator autonomously ordering a biopsy), the legal framework of malpractice begins to crumble. If a Total Agent misses a diagnosis because of a "multimodal conflict" between the EHR and the scan, who is at fault? The hospital that bought the agent? The developer who trained it? Or the radiologist who was "supervising" fifty agents at once? The transition to GMI requires a total overhaul of medical law, moving toward "Shared Liability" models that the legal system is currently ill-equipped to handle.

Summary: The Balance of Power

The future of Agentic GMI is a tightrope walk. We are building a system of immense power that can cure diseases at their inception and bring world-class care to the furthest corners of the globe. Yet, we must do so without losing the "Human Guardrail"—the skeptical, empathetic, and ultimately accountable physician.

The Future Outlook	The "Pro" (Opportunity)	The "Con" (Risk)
Diagnostic Power	Sub-visual, molecular detection.	"Logical" hallucinations that mislead experts.
Workforce	Liberates doctors for patient care.	Dangerous atrophy of manual diagnostic skills.
Access	Democratizes elite care globally.	Increases the "Cyber-Security" attack surface.
Ethical Framework	Hyper-personalized care pathways.	Massive concerns over data "colonization."

Conclusion: The Conductor's Final Note

The future of Agentic GMI is a tightrope walk. We are building a system that can cure diseases at their inception, yet we must do so without losing the Human Guardrail—the skeptical, empathetic, and ultimately accountable physician

CHAPTER 20: THE RENAISSANCE OF THE PHYSICIAN

As we close the blueprint for the agentic department of 2026 and look toward the decade beyond, we find ourselves at the end of a long-standing prophecy. For years, the narrative was one of replacement—the "End of Radiology" at the hands of silicon. Instead, we are witnessing a Renaissance.

The "Future Doctor" is not a master of the machine, nor its servant. They are the Ethical Anchor in a sea of autonomous data.

From "Image Reader" to "Information Architect"

In the pre-agentic era, a radiologist's value was determined by their eyes: their ability to spot a 3mm nodule on a 500-slice CT. In 2026, that task is handled by a background agent before the doctor even opens the file.

The Future Doctor's role has shifted from Perception to Synthesis.

- **The Clinical Nexus:** The doctor now spends their time connecting the "Agent's Findings" with the "Patient's Story." They are the ones who look at a high-confidence AI diagnosis and say, *"This doesn't match the patient's lived experience,"* providing the crucial final veto.

- **Managing the Ensemble:** A modern radiologist acts like a conductor. On a single case, they may oversee a Lung Agent, a Cardiac Agent, and a Liver Agent. Their expertise lies in resolving **the conflicts between** these agents to provide a unified, human-centric report.

The Three Pillars of the Future Physician

To thrive in the age of General Medical Intelligence (GMI), the 2030 physician relies on three skills that were rarely taught in 20th-century medical schools:

I. Probabilistic Literacy

The future doctor understands that "The AI says it's cancer" is a meaningless statement without understanding Precision and Recall. They are masters of the "p-value" and "confidence interval," knowing exactly when an agent's 92% certainty is actually a red flag for a "Logical Hallucination."

II. Algorithmic Empathy

As diagnostics become faster and more automated, the "Human Touch" becomes the most expensive and valuable commodity in healthcare. The future doctor uses the time "gifted" back by AI to engage in deep-dive consultations. They translate the cold, molecular logic of the agent into the warm, reassuring language of a healer.

III. Ethical Guardianship

The physician is the "Final Accountable Party." In a world of shared liability, the doctor is the ethical steward who ensures that the agentic system remains unbiased, transparent, and focused on the patient's dignity rather than just the hospital's throughput.

The New Education: Training the Pilot

Medical education has undergone a total "System Reset."

- **The AI Simulation Lab:** Residents no longer just look at static films. They are trained in "Stress Environments" where agents are intentionally biased or sabotaged (as discussed in Section IV), forcing the student to find the flaw.

- **Collaborative Boards:** Final exams (the "Boards" of 2030) test a student's ability to lead an AI-human team. A student fails not because they missed a finding, but because they failed to catch an agent's error.

Conclusion: The Shared Horizon

The "Agentic Department" is the final realization of the goal of medicine: to see what was previously invisible and to heal what was previously unreachable.

We are moving away from an era where a doctor was defined by what they knew, toward an era where they are defined by how they think. The machines have taken over the "Searching," but they have left the "Thinking" and the "Caring" entirely to us.

The rise of the agent is not the end of the doctor; it is the beginning of the Human Doctor.

EPILOGUE: THE QUIET REVOLUTION

It is a Tuesday morning in late 2026. Inside the headquarters of **Digi Health Services**, the air is quiet. There are no frantic sirens, no stacks of unread films, and no exhausted clinicians staring at monitors with blurred vision.

In this new reality, the "Agentic Department" has moved past the stage of novelty and into the realm of the invisible. Like the electricity that powers the hospital or the sterile air in the OR, the AI agents have become a fundamental, silent utility. They are the background pulse of modern medicine—constantly triaging, cross-referencing, and safeguarding every patient who walks through the door.

We began this journey by asking if a machine could replace a doctor. We end it with a different realization: the machine has actually revealed the doctor. By stripping away the hours of measurements, the repetitive data entry, and the administrative friction, we have uncovered the core of the medical profession that had been buried for decades.

The physician of 2026—the practitioner mentored by the vision of Dr. Basem Garada—is more human than ever. They have the time to sit with a patient, to explain a complex diagnosis without checking their watch, and to use their uniquely human intuition to solve the cases that even the most powerful General Medical Intelligence cannot crack.

The "Blueprint" provided in these pages is more than a technical manual; it is a social contract. It is a promise that as our technology grows more complex, our care will grow more personal.

The revolution did not happen with a bang or a grand replacement. It happened quietly, one agent at a time, until we woke up to find that we had finally built a healthcare system that works as fast as our pixels and as deeply as our hearts.

The scanners are ready. The agents are online. The future is in your hands.

EXECUTIVE SUMMARY: THE AGENTIC RADIOLOGY DEPARTMENT (2026–2030)

This summary encapsulates the strategic roadmap for transitioning from a traditional, modality-based radiology department to an Agentic Ecosystem. By 2026, AI agents have evolved from simple "tools" into autonomous "partners" capable of reasoning across clinical, imaging, and genomic data.

I. The Strategic Vision: From Pixels to Partners

In the 2026–2030 era, imaging is no longer a passive snapshot. It is a proactive diagnostic event.

- **The Orchestrator:** Every department is managed by a central "AI Orchestrator" that triages cases, pre-fetches historical data, and assigns specialized agents (Stroke, Oncology, Fracture) to each scan.
- **Multimodal Reasoning:** Agents no longer view images in a vacuum. They integrate **FHIR-based EHR data**, lab results, and real-time vitals to provide high-confidence, context-aware reports.
- **The Goal:** To reduce the "Time to Intervention" while increasing the "Cognitive Capacity" of the human radiologist.

II. Implementation Roadmap: The 7-Phase Lifecycle

Successful rollout requires a disciplined, modality-specific approach rather than a "plug-and-play" installation.

1. **Planning:** Identify high-friction "pain points" (e.g., ER backlogs) and define success KPIs.
2. **Development:** Fine-tune agents using local datasets to ensure performance matches specific scanner hardware.
3. **Testing (Shadow Mode):** Run agents in the background to validate accuracy against human "Gold Standard" reads without affecting live care.

4. **Production Rollout:** Phased integration starting with "AI-Assisted" documentation before moving to diagnostic support.

5. **Evaluation:** Continuous auditing of the **"AI Dividend"**—measuring gains in throughput, safety, and staff wellness.

6. **Administration:** Appointing **AI Stewards** to manage "Model Decay," security, and ethical guardrails.

7. **Upgrade:** Maintaining a modular tech stack (FHIR/DICOMweb) to allow for seamless model swaps as GMI (General Medical Intelligence) evolves.

III. The Future Balance: Pros vs. Cons

The Pros (Opportunities)	The Cons (Risks)
Precision: Sub-visual, molecular detection of Stage 1 disease.	**Hallucinations:** High-confidence, "logical" but incorrect AI reasoning.
Equity: Decentralized "AI-in-a-Box" pods bringing elite care to rural areas.	**Skill Atrophy:** Human loss of manual diagnostic skills due to over-reliance.
Efficiency: 80% reduction in documentation and administrative "drudgery."	**Liability:** Legal "Gray Zones" regarding autonomous machine decisions.
Humanity: Returning doctors to the bedside through "Time Recovery."	**Privacy:** Risks of "Data Colonization" by large-scale AI developers.

IV. Key Modality Takeaways

Modality	2026–2030 Strategic Focus	The "Agentic" Innovation
CT	High-Velocity Triage	**Zero-Latency Alerts:** Orchestrators prioritize life-critical cases (Stroke, PE, Hemorrhage) to the top of the worklist within milliseconds of scan completion.
X-Ray	Throughput & Accuracy	**Pre-exposure Positioning AI:** Computer vision agents give a "Green Light" for perfect patient positioning, reducing retake rates to near zero.
MRI	Scan Time Reduction	**Synthetic Sequence Generation:** Deep-learning reconstruction cuts scan times by **60–80%** while maintaining diagnostic texture and resolution.
Ultrasound	Operator Guidance	**Real-time Anatomical Mapping:** Agents provide "GPS-like" guidance for sonographers, auto-measuring organs and identifying missed spots in real-time.
Mammography	Screening Sensitivity	**5-Year Risk Prediction:** AI moves beyond detection to predictive analytics, assigning personalized risk scores to guide supplemental screening (MRI/US).
PET / SPECT	Molecular Precision	**Low-Tracer Synthesis:** Agents allow for diagnostic-quality imaging with **50% less radiopharmaceutical dose**, protecting patients and lowering costs.
Interventional	Real-time Navigation	**3D-Fusion Sterile HUD:** Voice-controlled agents overlay pre-op 3D maps onto live fluoroscopy, reducing "Total Fluoroscopy Time" and contrast use.

V. Final Conclusion: The New Social Contract

The rise of the Agentic Department does not herald the end of the radiologist. Instead, it marks the end of the radiologist as a "Data Entry Clerk."

By 2030, the radiologist is an Architect of Trust, providing the final ethical and clinical "veto" over a fleet of specialized agents. The machine provides the Calculation; the human provides the Compassion and Judgment. In this new era, we don't just see the disease; we see the patient through the lens of total, integrated intelligence.

GLOSSARY OF THE AGENTIC ERA

To wrap up your guide to the Agentic Radiology Department, this glossary serves as a technical and strategic reference for the terminology used throughout the text. These terms represent the intersection of clinical medicine, computer science, and administrative strategy in 2026.

A

- **Adversarial Attack:** A technique where subtle, often invisible "noise" is added to medical images to trick an AI agent into making a false diagnosis (e.g., hiding a tumor or creating a fake one).
- **Agentic AI:** AI systems that do not just process data but can reason, use tools, and take autonomous actions (like ordering a follow-up scan) based on a set of goals.
- **AI Dividend:** The measurable gain in time, money, or clinical outcomes achieved after the implementation of AI, often reinvested into patient care.
- **Automation Bias:** The human tendency to over-trust a machine's output, leading to the potential for a clinician to overlook an AI error.

B

- **Black Box Problem:** The lack of transparency in how deep-learning models reach a conclusion.
- **Bias Monitor:** An administrative tool that tracks AI performance across different demographics (race, age, gender) to ensure diagnostic equity.

C

- **Command Center:** The centralized hub of a 2026 radiology department where "Orchestrators" oversee the flow of AI-human workflows.
- **Contrastive Explanation:** A feature of Explainable AI where the agent explains why a finding is *Cancer* and specifically why it is *not* something else (like an infection).

D

- **DICOMweb:** The modern web-standard for exchanging medical images, allowing AI agents to query and retrieve scans via standard internet protocols.

- **Digital Twin:** A dynamic, virtual representation of a patient's unique physiology, created by integrating real-time imaging data, genomic markers, and longitudinal EHR records. In the Agentic Department, the Digital Twin is used by agents to run simulations—such as predicting how a specific tumor will respond to a radiotherapy plan—before the physical treatment begins.

F

- **FHIR (Fast Healthcare Interoperability Resources):** The global standard for exchanging electronic health records (EHR). It allows AI agents to "read" a patient's medical history.
- **Fusion Imaging:** The real-time overlay of two different modalities, such as placing a 3D MRI scan over a live 2D X-ray during surgery.

G

- **General Medical Intelligence (GMI):** The next evolution of AI that can reason across all medical modalities (imaging, blood work, genomics) simultaneously rather than focusing on one narrow task.

I

- **Incidentaloma:** A finding on a scan that is unrelated to the original reason for the test. AI agents are used to track these to ensure they are not lost to follow-up.

L

- **LMM (Large Multimodal Model):** An advanced AI architecture capable of processing and "reasoning" across multiple types of data simultaneously—such as DICOM images, clinical text, and laboratory values. Unlike traditional "Narrow AI" which can only look for one finding (e.g., a lung nodule), an LMM provides the holistic intelligence required for an Orchestrator Agent to understand a patient's entire clinical narrative.
- **LOINC (Logical Observation Identifiers Names and Codes):** A universal standard for identifying medical laboratory observations, used by AI to write structured reports.

M

- **MCP (Model Context Protocol):** A standard that allows different AI agents to share the "context" or "reasoning" of a case with one another.
- **Molecular Agent:** Programmable nanoparticles used in PET/SPECT that can "reason" at a cellular level to target specific tumors.

N

- **NTAP (New Technology Add-on Payment):** A reimbursement model where insurers provide extra payments for using advanced, FDA-cleared AI technology that improves outcomes.

O

- **Observation Resource:** The specific section of a FHIR record where an AI agent records its findings (measurements, risk scores, etc.).
- **Orchestrator:** The "brain" of the department—a primary AI agent that manages the workload, assigns specialized agents to cases, and alerts humans to emergencies.

P

- **Provenance:** In a medical record, the metadata that tracks exactly *who* (human or agent) authored a specific finding or measurement.

R

- **RAG (Retrieval-Augmented Generation):** A method where an AI agent "looks up" specific hospital guidelines or patient history before generating a diagnostic suggestion.

S

- **Shadow Mode:** A testing phase where a new AI agent runs in the background on live cases but its results are hidden from doctors until its accuracy is proven.
- **Sidecar Deployment:** A technical implementation where the AI runs alongside existing software without requiring a total system overhaul.
- **SUV (Standardized Uptake Value):** A mathematical measure of radiotracer concentration in PET scans, often automated by AI for precision.

X

- **XAI (Explainable AI):** AI designed to "show its work" using heatmaps or logic trees so that a human radiologist can verify its reasoning.

FURTHER READING & REFERENCES

This section provides the intellectual and technical scaffolding upon which the Agentic Department is built. For the practitioner or executive looking to dive deeper into the mechanics of the transition, the following resources are recommended.

I. Core Technical Standards

- **HL7 FHIR (Fast Healthcare Interoperability Resources):** The global standard for exchanging electronic health records. By 2026, it is the primary bridge allowing AI agents to pull real-time clinical context (labs, medications, and social determinants) into their diagnostic reasoning.
  - *Reference:* HL7 FHIR Specification (v5.0.0)
- **DICOMweb™:** The RESTful implementation of the DICOM standard. It enables web-based AI microservices to query (QIDO-RS), retrieve (WADO-RS), and store (STOW-RS) imaging data using standard web protocols rather than heavy legacy VPNs.
  - *Reference:* DICOM PS3.18: Web Services
- **Model Context Protocol (MCP):** Introduced by Anthropic in late 2024 and standardized throughout 2025, MCP is the "USB-C for AI." It provides a secure, universal interface that allows LLMs to interact with medical data silos and tools (like PACS or EHRs) without custom integration for every vendor.
  - *Reference:* Model Context Protocol Specification

II. Strategic & Ethical Frameworks

- **NIST AI Risk Management Framework (AI RMF 1.0):** The definitive guide for managing risks to individuals and organizations. In 2025, healthcare-specific extensions (such as those from *Censinet*) have become the gold standard for auditing bias and security in autonomous agents.
  - *Reference:* NIST AI RMF 1.0 (NIST AI 100-1)
- **The 2025 Physician Sentiment Survey (Athenahealth):** A critical study on the "AI Dividend," showing how ambient AI and agentic documentation have led to a **10% decrease in physician burnout** by automating administrative "pajama time."
  - *Reference:* Athenahealth 2025 Physician Sentiment Survey

- **The Algorithmic Empathy Manifesto:** While a conceptual framework, it aligns with recent 2025 literature (e.g., *Philips Future Health Index 2025*) regarding the need to close the "Trust Gap" between patients and AI-driven diagnostics through human-AI partnership.

III. Recommended Literature & Academic Foundations

- **"Explainable AI (XAI) in Medical Imaging" (2025):** Recent studies in the *Journal of Medical Internet Research (JMIR)* and *Frontiers in Digital Health* highlight how techniques like Grad-CAM and SHAP values are moving AI from "black box" to transparent partner.
    - *Key Paper:* "Explainable Artificial Intelligence-Driven Analysis of Radiology Reports" (JMIR, Oct 2025).

- **"Digital Twins for Personalized Medicine" (2025):** Research published in *Nature Digital Medicine* and *Frontiers* details how digital replicas of patients are now achieving 97% accuracy in predicting disease progression (e.g., Alzheimer's tissue loss) years before symptoms appear.
    - *Reference:* Digital Twins in Healthcare: A Comprehensive Review (Frontiers, 2025)

- **"Reasoning Over Perception":** Academic shift toward Large Multimodal Models (LMMs) that use chain-of-thought reasoning to explain *why* they flagged a finding, rather than just drawing a box around a pixel.

IV. Key Academic & Technical References

1. Multi-Step Clinical Reasoning (The "Thinking Mode")

- **"Capabilities of GPT-5 on Multimodal Medical Reasoning" (arXiv, 2025):** This study evaluates the newest LMMs as "generalist multimodal reasoners." It demonstrates how these models use zero-shot Chain-of-Thought to outperform earlier versions (like GPT-4o) in visual question answering, moving from simple perception to expert-level diagnostic support.

- **"Benchmarking the Thinking Mode of Multimodal Large Language Models in Clinical Tasks" (arXiv, Nov 2025):** This research distinguishes between the "non-thinking" (immediate output) and "thinking mode" (explicit internal reasoning). It notes that as medical tasks increase in complexity, activating the reasoning process is essential for reliability.

2. Multimodal Chain-of-Thought (MCoT)

- **"Multimodal Chain-of-Thought Reasoning: A Comprehensive Survey" (ResearchGate/ACL, 2025):** This systematic survey defines MCoT as the integration of CoT with multimodal models. It highlights how these models address unique challenges in healthcare by creating human-like, step-by-step processes for 3D and structured data.

- **"Medical Chain-of-Thought Reasoning" (Emergent Mind, Oct 2025):** This resource details frameworks like DR-CoT (Diagnostic Reasoning CoT) and MedCodex. These frameworks enforce clinical protocols—such as summarizing evidence, ranking differentials, and proposing follow-up questions—mirroring real-life physician workflows.

3. Shift in Architecture: From "Siloed" to "Integrated"

- **"Large Language Models and Large Multimodal Models in Medical Imaging: A Primer for Physicians" (Journal of Nuclear Medicine, 2025):** This primer explains how LMMs act as "Cognitive Engines." Instead of being trained for one specific task (like bone age), they use pre-trained reasoning capabilities to navigate the entire multimodal ecosystem of radiology.

- **"Multimodal Large Language Models in Medical Imaging: Current State and Future Directions" (PMC, Dec 2025):** This review emphasizes the move toward "Region-Grounded Reasoning," where model outputs are explicitly linked to specific image coordinates, effectively explaining the "perception" through a "reasoning" narrative.

THE FUTURE OF RADIOLOGY IS AGENTIC.

We are standing at the threshold of a new era in healthcare. By 2026, Artificial Intelligence has evolved from a passive tool into an active, reasoning partner. In *The Agentic Department*, **Dr. Basem Garada** provides the definitive strategic blueprint for navigating this transition.

This book is not just about technology—it is about the integration of human judgment with machine intelligence. Spanning the entire implementation lifecycle across seven critical modalities, Dr. Garada outlines how to build a department where AI agents handle the calculation, allowing physicians to focus on what matters most: compassion, judgment, and complex care.

Within these pages, you will discover:

- **The 7-Phase Implementation Lifecycle:** A step-by-step roadmap for deploying AI across CT, MRI, Ultrasound, X-Ray, PET, SPECT, and Interventional Radiology.
- **General Medical Intelligence (GMI):** How the next generation of multimodal AI will bridge the gap between imaging, genomics, and electronic health records.
- **Clinical Team Dynamics:** Detailed roles for Radiologists, Technologists, and Nurses in an agent-augmented environment.
- **The Strategic Future:** An honest evaluation of the pros and cons—from hyper-personalized precision to the challenges of algorithmic bias and skill atrophy.

Digi Health Services is proud to present this essential guide for hospital executives, clinical leads, and futurists ready to lead the charge into the next decade of medical excellence.

ABOUT THE AUTHOR

Dr. Basem Garada is a visionary leader in medical imaging, digital health, and the architect of the "Agentic Blueprint" for modern radiology. As the founder and principal of Digi Health Services, he operates at the high-stakes intersection of clinical practice, artificial intelligence, and systems engineering.

With a career dedicated to bridging the gap between legacy hospital infrastructure and the future of autonomous care, Dr. Garada has become a sought-after advisor for departments worldwide. His work focuses on transforming traditional "volume-based" imaging centers into self-optimizing, agentic ecosystems—environments where technology does not just assist the physician but actively collaborates to improve patient outcomes.

A Legacy of Innovation

Dr. Garada's expertise is rooted in a deep understanding of the "Triple-A" framework: Administrative efficiency, AI-technical integration, and Anatomical/Clinical accuracy. He is a leading proponent of:

- **Explainable AI (XAI)**: Moving the industry away from "Black Box" algorithms toward transparent reasoning chains that clinicians can trust.

- **Operational Excellence**: Leveraging the "AI Dividend" to restore physician wellness and eliminate the administrative drudgery that leads to burnout.

- **Global Health Equity**: Pioneering the use of "AI-in-a-Box" and GMI (General Medical Intelligence) to democratize elite-level diagnostic expertise in underserved regions.

The Digi Health Vision

Through Digi Health Services, Dr. Garada provides the strategic and technical "scaffolding" necessary for health systems to survive and thrive in the 2026–2030 era. His approach is defined by the belief that the rise of the machine is not the end of the doctor, but the beginning of a Physician Renaissance—one where the human provides the compassion and ethical judgment, while the agent provides the precision and speed.

www.ingramcontent.com/pod-product-compliance
Ingram Content Group UK Ltd.
Pitfield, Milton Keynes, MK11 3LW, UK
UKHW062012041026
15591UKWH00017B/1303

9 798994 956533